"In this work Kathryn Rickard explores surrender as a living process, staying close to moments of experience as they unfold. She shows how something in us loosens and begins to come alive in ways that cannot be forced, opening pathways into deeper contact with ourselves and others."

**Michael Eigen**, *PhD, author of* Contact with the Depths, The Sensitive Self, and The Psychoanalytic Mystic; *psychoanalyst*

"Surrender is often seen as defeat, but Rickard shows that it can unleash our greatest successes. With the serenity to accept what cannot be changed, we gain the will to face our options knowingly, openly, and intentionally. Pairing meticulous theory with in-depth case studies, Rickard offers a clear playbook of directed risk and openness that leads to genuine psychological transformation."

**Richard Granger**, *PhD, author of* Big Brain: The Origins and Future of Human Intelligence; *professor, Dartmouth College; director, Brain Engineering Laboratory*

"Kathryn Rickard has written a much-needed volume on the critical psychoanalytic construct of surrender—a term too infrequently discussed and rarely understood. Her timely effort to elucidate surrender is especially laudable... This work fills an essential niche in the psychotherapeutic and psychoanalytic literature. Beautifully written in accessible language, it is a gift to both psychoanalytic and lay communities. A must-read."

**Melvin E. Miller**, *PhD, co-editor of* Spirituality, Ethics, and Relationship in Adulthood: Clinical and Theoretical Explorations; *Charles Dana professor of Psychology, Emeritus, Norwich University; Psychoanalyst*

# The Psychoanalytic Anatomy of Surrender

*The Psychoanalytic Anatomy of Surrender* offers an original psychoanalytic model of surrender, illuminating how the inner structures that inhibit aliveness may gradually loosen through emotional experience, therapeutic work, and psychological transformation.

Through detailed clinical case studies and original theoretical contributions, the book explores surrender as a psychological process unfolding across multiple dimensions of emotional life—from rigidity, defensiveness, and control toward greater receptivity, love, gratitude, wisdom, and deeper engagement with lived experience. Integrating psychoanalysis with philosophy and broader contemplative traditions, Rickard develops a practical framework for understanding psychological transformation in both patients and therapists.

Written for psychoanalysts, psychotherapists, scholars, and psychologically minded readers, this book offers a clinical and conceptual language for understanding surrender and its role in therapeutic growth, emotional development, and psychological aliveness.

**Kathryn Rickard**, Psy.D., is a clinical psychologist, psychoanalytic practitioner, and author with over two decades of clinical experience. Her work focuses on the conditions under which emotional experience can be encountered, avoided, or sustained within the analytic setting. *The Psychoanalytic Anatomy of Surrender* expands upon her original research exploring surrender as a psychological process within psychoanalytic treatment.

# The Psychoanalytic Anatomy of Surrender

## Breaking Through the Inner Structures that Inhibit Aliveness

**Kathryn Rickard**

Routledge
Taylor & Francis Group
LONDON AND NEW YORK

Designed cover image: Getty Images

First published 2027
by Routledge
4 Park Square, Milton Park, Abingdon, Oxon OX14 4RN

and by Routledge
605 Third Avenue, New York, NY 10158

*Routledge is an imprint of the Taylor & Francis Group, an Informa business*



*British Library Cataloguing in Publication Data*
A catalogue record for this book is available from the British Library

ISBN: 9781041350552 (hbk)
ISBN: 9781041340508 (pbk)
ISBN: 9781003795803 (ebk)

DOI: 10.4324/9781003795803

Typeset in Optima
by Taylor & Francis Books

For all the surrender opportunities—beautiful, painful, and occasionally operating under dubious management—that found me.

To some I leapt; others I initially resisted with considerable enthusiasm.

The education, while unorthodox, appears to have worked.

# Contents

# Table

# Acknowledgments

This book took shape gradually over many years. Its ideas matured through sustained analytic study, clinical immersion, and the discipline of returning repeatedly to a phenomenon that resisted easy resolution. What follows reflects a continuity of attention rather than a single moment of insight.

Although the thinking in these pages is my own, it has been shaped by conversations, challenges, and remarks that proved more consequential than they initially appeared. I am particularly indebted to one analyst whose thinking influenced my own and who, at a pivotal moment, observed that I had not yet surrendered—despite what I experienced at the time as significant external sacrifice. I resisted that claim. The irritation it provoked exposed a confusion that required further examination. That challenge remained and ultimately sharpened the inquiry that became this book.

I am equally grateful to the patients who entrusted me with the unfolding of their inner worlds. Their willingness to remain with confusion, repetition, dread, gratitude, and love made this model possible. Whatever coherence the work achieves rests upon their seriousness and courage.

I am also grateful to Kate Hawes at Routledge for recognizing the project and supporting its development.

# Author's Preface

Some readers approach experience by looking—and continuing to look—without requiring it to resolve too quickly. This stance is not common. It depends on a tolerance for uncertainty, and a capacity to remain with what does not immediately organize itself into meaning.

It is within this stance that surrender becomes possible.

Surrender. The word sits oddly in the mouth—heavy, often misunderstood. It is commonly equated with failure, with giving up, with a relinquishing of strength. But this misrecognition obscures its psychological function. Surrender is not collapse, but a form of letting go—a shift in how experience is held, no longer organized solely around control. It requires a movement toward what cannot be fully managed or predicted, and for that reason is often resisted.

When Simone Biles withdrew from the Tokyo Olympics in 2021, the moment was widely interpreted through the language of strength or failure. She described a loss of coordination between mind and body, an inability to orient herself in space, and a recognition that continuing would not be safe. What she enacted can be understood as a form of surrender—not the collapse of will, but its suspension.

Rather than adhering to a cultural script that prioritizes performance at any cost, she turned inward and allowed that internal signal to determine action. The gesture was brief, but structurally significant: a relinquishing of imposed direction in favor of contact with something more immediate and less organized, where action is no longer driven by expectation but reorganized around what can actually be sustained.

That moment struck something in me. Not because it was rare, but because it was so rarely allowed. Surrender continues to be misrecognized—conflated with failure, passivity, or indulgence, and therefore resisted even when it becomes necessary. What appeared in that moment was something else: not a collapse of agency, but a reorganization of it—a turning inward that allowed action to follow from a different point of contact, one not governed by performance or control.

Surrender does not always take the form of stillness. At times, it appears as movement into action—when resistance to what one is called to do can no longer be sustained. This may involve stepping into something difficult or unwanted: speaking when one would prefer to remain silent, assuming responsibility when withdrawal would feel easier, or acting in the presence of fear without first resolving it. In such moments, the shift is not toward passivity, but toward alignment with what has already begun to press forward. What defines surrender is not the direction of movement, but a change in the relation to experience from which that movement emerges—no longer organized around avoidance, but around contact with what cannot be deferred.

That image of surrender did not begin for me in the therapy room. It began in childhood—reading about mystics, saints, and seekers who, in moments of rupture, relinquished certainty and moved toward something less defined but more compelling. I was drawn to their language—not because I understood it, but because it carried a current of truth I could not yet name but felt compelled to follow.

Religion does not structure my clinical work. What draws me to mystical texts is not doctrine, but the precision with which they describe interior experience. My connection to these traditions is private and symbolic, engaged less as belief than as a way of remaining in contact with forms of experience that exceed ordinary conceptual language.

This book emerges from that curiosity. It began with research into Focusing-Oriented Psychotherapy, where I sought a language for the subtle, often ineffable process of inner yielding. In a brief correspondence, Eugene Gendlin clarified that his model was not grounded in mystical frameworks, nor intended to describe surrender in the way I had begun to understand it. The therapy transcripts were rich, but they did not account for certain moments—moments of letting go that were not quite insight, not quite catharsis, but something less easily named.

To deepen the analytic work, I turned to mystical texts—not for their conclusions, but for their capacity to articulate experience at the limits of understanding. These writings offered metaphors, rhythms, and distinctions that illuminated what was unfolding beneath the surface of therapeutic change. The convergence of these sources—clinical material and centuries-old reflections on inner life—gave form to what I came to understand as the surrender process.

Later, I began to recognize it in the consulting room—moments in which patients, often haltingly, began to relinquish control. Not because they were instructed to, but because something in them could no longer maintain the effort required not to.

I moved from Canada to the United States in my late twenties—more than 3,000 miles from home, without a clear plan, established footing, or reliable structure to return to. It was not a calculated decision, nor one grounded in certainty. It was a form of surrender: a movement into uncertainty, guided less by confidence than by the sense that something essential required engagement, even without an assurance of outcome.

In Canada, psychotherapy often remained understated, shaped by a quiet but persistent stigma that limited its visibility in everyday discourse. In the United States, it carried greater cultural permission and presence, but not always a corresponding depth of psychological inquiry. Between these contexts, a set of questions began to take shape: what makes surrender possible, and what makes it intolerable? Why does it emerge in some moments and not in others, even when the conditions appear similar? And what determines whether an individual can remain in contact with what surrender exposes?

In clinical work, the persistence of avoidance becomes increasingly evident. Patients remain organized around what is familiar, even when that familiarity constrains them and limits the range of experience available to them. Letting go can register not only as uncertainty, but as a form of psychic loss, and is therefore guarded against with considerable force. Surrender cannot be produced through effort alone, nor does it respond to intention in any direct way. It does not emerge through instruction, but through shifts in how experience is held, tolerated, and engaged. The analytic task is not to induce surrender, but to establish the conditions under which it becomes possible without forcing its arrival.

I do not approach surrender as a goal, nor as a technique to be implemented or applied. It is not something to be achieved, but something that becomes recognizable as it begins to take form within the analytic process. What is offered here is not a method, but a way of observing the conditions under which such shifts occur—how contact deepens, how resistance reorganizes itself in response to that contact, and how new forms of experience become available without being imposed.

This book traces the psychoanalytic anatomy of surrender: the structures that support it, the defenses that inhibit it, and the conditions under which it emerges. It is an attempt to map what can be observed while remaining in contact with what resists full articulation or premature definition. At its center is a question: what allows experience to move beyond the structures that constrain it, without collapsing under the strain of that movement? Surrender does not resolve that question, but alters the conditions under which it can be encountered and sustained.

# Introduction

## The Model, the Map, and the Psychoanalytic Anatomy of Surrender

Surrender is an experience that often goes unrecognized, even as it shapes some of the most consequential moments of psychic life. It escapes notice not because it is rare, but because it does not announce itself. It appears in shifts that do not register as decisions: when insistence gives way, when tension softens, when something previously held is released. These moments are not typically marked as events. They register instead as a change in relation to experience—less organized around control, more open to what is occurring.

At the same time, surrender is often resisted. For some, psychic life becomes organized around the effort to control and contain experience, avoiding forms of contact that feel destabilizing or unmanageable. In such conditions, aliveness becomes constrained—not absent, but limited in how fully it can be registered or sustained.

By aliveness, I don't mean a generic sense of wellness or affect regulation—I mean the felt inner movement toward vitality, contact, meaning, and presence. To surrender to aliveness is to attune to one's internal signals—sensations, impulses, intuitions, emotions—as they arise, allowing them to register, inform, and guide. It is the capacity to let inner life shape perception rather than bypass or rearrange it to meet outer expectations. Simone Weil observed that attention is bound up not with the will but with desire—more precisely, with consent. In this context, aliveness is not merely the presence of sensation or emotion, but the act of receiving one's experience with that kind of attention—undistracted, receptive, and open to being changed by what it encounters. In this sense, aliveness does not refer to the intensity of experience, but to the capacity to remain in contact with it as it unfolds.

As the surrender process deepens, we encounter concepts that are rarely explored in depth within traditional psychoanalytic literature. These capacities—such as *Non-Willing, Ecstasy,* and *Emergent Relationship*—often extend beyond the boundaries of psychoanalytic discourse into realms more commonly explored by mystics and spiritual traditions. In the original development of this surrender model, exemplary mystical texts provided a framework for understanding these deeper states of letting go. These texts

DOI: 10.4324/9781003795803-1

offered rich language and insight into experiences of profound release and unity that are less frequently addressed in psychological contexts.

The configurations described in this model are presented sequentially for clarity, but they do not constitute a fixed progression. They refer to forms of psychological organization that emerge, recede, and reorganize under particular internal and relational conditions. Clinical observation suggests that movement among them is variable and nonlinear, with patients returning to earlier configurations under altered conditions of contact. What appears as repetition may therefore reflect not stasis, but a change in how experience is held and engaged.

This book seeks to expand that initial framework through a more explicit engagement with psychoanalytic principles and therapeutic application. While the original model drew upon mystical texts to illuminate the deepest movements of surrender, the present work develops these insights within the language and practice of psychoanalysis. As Albert Einstein once remarked, "The most beautiful experience we can have is the mysterious. It is the fundamental emotion that stands at the cradle of true art and true science."[1] Surrender requires us to tolerate this sense of mystery—to release our need for certainty and venture into the unknown regions of the self. The mystical thus serves as the original basis, while the work here represents a psychoanalytic expansion, examining surrender not only as a process within the patient but as a dynamic that also unfolds within the therapist. By grounding these advanced capacities in psychoanalytic language, the model becomes a kind of anatomical atlas—a bridge between the psychological and the transcendent, mapping the inner terrain of surrender in ways that make it both observable and livable.

This book is called *The Psychoanalytic Anatomy of Surrender*, but not in the way anatomy is typically imagined. What follows is not a dissection of a dead process, but a mapping of a living one—full of breath, tension, rupture, and repair. This is not the body pinned open; it's the psyche mid-motion. We are not asking what surrender is. We're asking how it moves.

Unlike many books on transformation that emphasize active self-improvement, resilience, or 'pushing through' difficulties, *The Psychoanalytic Anatomy of Surrender* takes a different approach. It highlights surrender as an essential, often misunderstood psychological process. True transformation emerges not through force but through the ability to let go, break down, and yield to unconscious shifts that cannot be willed into being. Surrender also bears on the capacity to think beyond rigid organization, particularly in contexts where polarized forms of understanding dominate. By relinquishing rigid control, individuals can open themselves to new perspectives, fostering adaptability and deeper understanding.

## On Hitting Rock Bottom

Not all surrender unfolds gradually. Sometimes it is preceded by sudden rupture, collapse, or what is often called hitting rock bottom. These moments are not the same as surrender, but they can create the conditions for it. Collapse is not yet transformation, but it may mark the failure of a psychic structure that once held things together.

In the language of this book, these moments often mark the breaking point of the *Closed* state—the moment when rigid defenses no longer work, and the psyche becomes exposed to something it cannot metabolize alone. What follows is not always progress; it may be chaos, retreat, or silence. But it can also be the beginning of movement—toward dependency, regression, or the capacity to tolerate something previously unbearable. Surrender, in these moments, is not willed. It emerges from contact with what can no longer be denied. The therapeutic task is not to offer insight too quickly, but to stay present with what is raw, disoriented, or newly exposed. From here, symbolic life may begin to form—but only if the atmosphere can hold it.

Rooted in psychoanalytic theory, this book moves beyond the language of self-help and quick-fix frameworks. Drawing on real clinical cases, it offers a nuanced exploration of unconscious resistance, defensive structures, and the conditions necessary for genuine surrender. While many writings on surrender emerge from spiritual traditions, *The Psychoanalytic Anatomy of Surrender* integrates these mystical foundations with a rigorous psychoanalytic lens—making the process more clinically applicable and emotionally precise.

Another distinctive feature of this book is its dual perspective: it examines surrender not only in the patient but also in the therapist. The therapeutic relationship is itself a site of surrender, requiring both parties to navigate vulnerability, uncertainty, and trust. This book treats surrender as a dynamic interplay, one that unfolds between therapist and patient and shapes the depth and effectiveness of the therapeutic work.

Furthermore, *The Psychoanalytic Anatomy of Surrender* is grounded in original research, expanding on an academic model first developed during the author's graduate studies (Rickard, 2008). Rather than treating surrender as an abstract construct, the book examines how it emerges within analytic work, through close attention to clinical process. One of psychoanalysis' enduring discoveries is that the mind reveals itself not only through what it can express, but through the forms of experience it cannot yet permit. Resistance, distortion, silence, and partial contact are therefore not merely obstacles to inquiry, but disclosures of the psychic organization through which surrender must pass. Surrender is not approached as a generalized human experience, but as something that takes form under specific relational and psychological conditions, often marked by resistance, distortion, or partial contact.

Although the model is derived from psychoanalytic practice, the movements it describes are not confined to the consulting room. Surrender may be encountered under conditions of emotional intensity, relational exposure, or psychological rupture—situations in which previously established ways of organizing experience no longer hold. What distinguishes these moments is not their content, but the demand they place on the individual's capacity to remain in contact with what is unfolding without immediate resolution.

In analytic work, this may take the form of acknowledging dependency within the transference, remaining with affect that had previously been avoided, or recognizing aspects of the self that had not been taken up as one's own. Across contexts, surrender is not defined by what is experienced, but by a change in the individual's relation to that experience as it emerges.

## The Humans Who Carry the Work

The people you'll meet in this book are not simply case studies; they reflect different ways in which surrender is resisted, feared, or approached within psychic life. Each encounters it under particular conditions—through hesitation, avoidance, or partial contact—as something begins to give way in how experience is held. Their identities have been carefully altered to protect confidentiality, but their emotional truths remain intact, drawn from real clinical experiences.

While no single account can encompass the full range of cultural, social, and familial experience, the focus here remains on the organization of the inner world. Defensive structures, patterns of avoidance, and repetitions of relational experience take different forms across contexts, but the underlying dynamics of how experience is resisted or allowed into contact remain structurally recognizable. Cultural and familial conditions shape how surrender is approached, feared, or disavowed, but they do not determine its possibility.

The characters in this book illuminate how surrender unfolds—or doesn't—primarily within a Western framework shaped by cultural values like independence and control. But the model itself is not bound to that perspective. It's meant to reflect something more universal: the way all human beings resist, approach, and sometimes allow surrender.

These humans did not simply illustrate the process. Their sessions, dreams, resistances, and breakthroughs gave the model shape. Through their stories, we explore what makes surrender feel impossible, what allows it to happen, and what it asks of us in the deeper work of transformation.

### *Gabriella*

Gabriella lives alone. She keeps the place neat—nothing excessive, nothing out of order. There are a few framed photos, mostly from years ago. She dusts them regularly, though she rarely stops to look.

She was a teacher for many years. The kind who stayed late without being asked. Parents trusted her. Colleagues relied on her to cover things quietly.

She was known for being steady. "You can always count on Gabriella," one of them once said, and it stuck. It felt accurate. Safer that way.

She still keeps in touch with a former colleague—cards at the holidays, the occasional message to check in. They exchange small updates. Nothing that lingers too long. It's enough to maintain contact without having to enter it.

If she needs something, she tends to let it pass. The thought appears, then folds back in on itself. It is easier to manage things on her own. Less risk of getting it wrong.

When she was younger, she tried at times to say more. She remembers the feeling of it building—something she wanted to express, though she couldn't always name it. Her mother would grow tense before she had finished speaking, as if anticipating something unwelcome. Then the shift—her voice sharper, final. Gabriella learned to feel it coming and to stop before it arrived.

Her father was easier to be with. He did not interrupt. But when she spoke, he would listen in a way that didn't quite land. A nod, a brief acknowledgment, and then his attention would drift. She remembers noticing it, even then, and adjusting. Shortening what she said. Keeping things contained.

Over time, it became less clear what she might have said if she hadn't needed to manage it.

Therapy is new to her. She wasn't sure what she was looking for exactly. "Nothing's wrong," she said at first. "I just thought... maybe it would be good to talk."

Don't lean too far. Don't let go of too much.

### *Winston*

Winston has known for a long time that something is not right, though he would not put it that way. Not to himself. Not to anyone.

His house isn't empty, but it might as well be. There are people there—people he barely knows, people who drift in and out, people who need a place to sleep. He doesn't tell them to leave. He doesn't ask questions. The dishes pile up, the floor stays unswept, his reflection in the bathroom mirror is something he avoids.

His job still exists, just barely. He still shows up, just barely. He has a sense of how close things are to giving way, though he doesn't say it out loud.

His father was a surgeon.

His father did not tolerate things going off track. Winston remembers the way he would correct small details—how something was set down, how something was said—until it matched what he expected. It wasn't loud. It didn't need to be.

His mother adjusted around it. She kept things even, smoothing over moments before they turned. Later, Winston would notice her glass refilled, though he hadn't seen her pour it.

Winston became a doctor as well, though not in the same way. A general practitioner. Easy to overlook.

Sex happens. It doesn't seem to matter much. Men, women, strangers—brief encounters that end as quickly as they begin.

He did not resist coming to therapy, though he would not describe himself as needing help. "Things could be better," he said at one point, and left it there.

### *Bill*

The machines don't ask much of him. They don't need anything. That's what he likes about them. You turn them on, they do what they're supposed to do. If something's off, you fix it. Simple.

The military was like that too. Clear. Structured. You learned your part and did it well. He was good at it. Better than most. He still thinks about it sometimes—how things ran, how you knew where you stood.

Now he works long shifts. Same place, same route home. He'll stop for gas, sometimes pick up a six-pack without really deciding to. The house is quiet when he gets in. His wife is usually in the other room, the television on. They'll talk a little—what needs to get done, what's coming up. Then it tapers off.

The marriage holds. It's been that way for a while. Nothing in particular is wrong. Nothing much changes either.

He drinks most nights. Not enough to cause trouble. Enough to take the edge off, if there is one.

Therapy wasn't his idea exactly. Someone mentioned it. He didn't see a reason not to come.

He sits, answers when he's asked something, leaves when the hour is up.

### *Jerome*

Jerome is meticulous. Controlled. Always prepared. He knows how to make a case—how to lay something out so it holds together, how to anticipate where it might come apart.

His mother used to tell him to be careful. Not in a dramatic way. Just often enough that it stayed with him. Don't let people in too easily. She worked hard, expected the same from him, and did not have much patience for things that got in the way.

He learned to keep things in order. School, work, relationships—each had its place. He speaks clearly, directly, rarely more than necessary. People tend to take him seriously.

He built a life that works. Stable. Accounted for. Nothing left exposed if it can be helped.

Lately, though, something has begun to press in—not in a way he would describe as a problem exactly, but enough that it is harder to ignore.

He came to therapy after noticing that his usual ways of managing things were requiring more effort and were no longer producing the same result.

### *Tinsley*

She knows how to present well. It's a skill.

She calls herself a Creative Consultant. Most of her work lives online—images, language, a version of things that holds together if you don't look too closely. She is good at it. At finding the angle that fits.

At home, things were less consistent. What was right one day could be wrong the next. She learned to track the shifts, to adjust quickly enough to stay in place.

She was told she was special. It was understood more than said outright. The world outside didn't respond the same way. School, work—things would start, then stop. People misunderstood her, or she lost interest. It was rarely clear which.

Relationships followed a similar pattern. She was drawn to women who needed something—attention, stability, direction. It worked, for a time. Then something would change. They would pull away, or turn on her, or leave. That part stayed with her.

Therapy is no exception. She watches closely. Listens for inconsistencies. Waits for the moment something doesn't quite hold.

She hasn't said what she wants from it.

### *On Character Placement Across Capacities*

Not every character appears in every chapter. Each patient's surrender process unfolds differently—some develop access to a range of capacities, while others stall, regress, or transform in more subtle ways. For example, Bill's surrender remains largely limited at the level of the *Closed* capacity, though he may show minor signs of movement later. Tinsley, too, resists deeper surrender, retreating into control and projection. Their limited appearances reflect the reality that not all patients develop or sustain access to every capacity of surrender, nor do these capacities emerge in a fixed order. This was an intentional choice, meant to reflect the non-linear and varied nature of real psychological work.

## Overview of the Chapters

Each chapter takes up a different configuration of surrender as it appears in analytic work—its resistances, hesitations, loosening, and reorganization. Together, they form an anatomy that is not sequential but relational, organized less as a path to be followed than as a field in which different forms of contact become possible under particular conditions.

This book approaches surrender as a capacity that develops within the analytic process. Drawing on psychoanalytic theory, clinical encounters, and lived experience, it considers surrender not as passivity, but as an active psychological movement—one that requires contact, endurance, and the gradual loosening of established forms of organization. At the center of this work is a model of surrender in psychotherapy, developed through graduate research and extended across two decades of clinical practice, which traces the conditions under which deeper contact with one's inner world becomes possible.

In a world increasingly shaped by rigidity, polarization, and the demand for control, the capacity to surrender takes on renewed significance. What follows examines the psychological structures that support or inhibit this capacity. Like the body's regulatory systems, these processes—dependency, containment, regression, and tolerance of frustration—must function in relation to one another for deeper transformation to occur.

The chart that follows offers a view of this anatomy. As with any living system, these structures are interdependent, less like steps in a sequence than elements in dynamic relation within a shared field. Some strengthen others, some recede, and some remain latent until conditions allow them to emerge. As the chapters unfold, these configurations come into view through clinical material, each patient revealing a different arrangement of what holds, what collapses, and what, when allowed to move, brings a sense of aliveness.

## Configurations Within the Surrender Model

### *Chart Overview*

If the foundational configurations are the vital organs of the psyche, the deepening capacities function as its integrative systems—organizing meaning, regulating emotional metabolism, and enabling connection. The transformational capacities, then, function like the organism's highest capacities: they circulate new insight, release internal blockages, and prepare the self for integration at the level of love and wisdom. But even these are challenged at the farthest edge—*A Nameless Dread*—where the psyche confronts dissolution and rebuilds through surrender.

## A Note on the Structure of the Model

As this book develops and expands my original surrender model in light of clinical experience, some chapters include brief justification sections explaining the placement or inclusion of particular configurations, especially where the model has been revised since its earliest form. These are not formal arguments but reflections: thoughts on why certain psychological capacities or preconditions—often felt more than named in the therapeutic field—deserve recognition as distinct structures in the psychoanalytic anatomy of surrender.

Some of these first emerged through mystical texts, where language reached beyond the clinical. Others revealed themselves gradually, in the

*Table 1* Experiential configurations in the psychoanalytic field of surrender

| *Domain of the Surrender Process* | *Experiential Configuration* | *Illustrative Clinical Process* | *Anatomical Function (Metaphor)* |
|---|---|---|---|
| Foundational Configurations | | | |
| | Closed | Defensive organization dominates; surrender experienced as threat | Organs of Psychic Survival (Foundational Capacities) |
| | Capacity to Depend | Development of trust in relation to another mind | |
| | Open-Ended Attention | Sustaining contact with experience without premature organization | |
| | Capacity to Regress | Allowing earlier emotional states to emerge within analytic safety | |
| Releasement: Initial Movements (Level A) | | | |
| | Capacity to Contain | Holding experience until thought becomes possible | Integrative Systems (e.g. Symbolic Digestion, Psychic Metabolism) |
| | Readiness for Anxiety | Increasing tolerance for uncertainty | |
| | Capacity to Accept Reality | Recognizing reality without defensive distortion | |
| | Frustration Tolerance | Remaining in contact with emotional difficulty | |
| | Capacity to Symbolize | Transforming experience into images and thought | |

| *Domain of the Surrender Process* | *Experiential Configuration* | *Illustrative Clinical Process* | *Anatomical Function (Metaphor)* |
|---|---|---|---|
| | Subjective Appropriation | Owning emotional experience as one's own | |
| | Discipline Not to Reason | Suspending explanatory control over experience | |
| | Suffering Necessary for Transformation | Remaining with destabilizing psychic experience | |
| | Purification (Catharsis) | Clearing defensive distortions from experience | |
| | Preparation for Love | Recognizing the other as separate | |
| Releasement: Relinquishment of Control (Level B) | | | |
| | Non-Willing | Letting go of deliberate psychological control | Neural and Affective Repatterning Systems |
| | Emergent Relationship | Relational awareness begins structuring experience | |
| | Ecstasy | Expanded contact with psychic experience | |
| | Doubt | Loosening certainty and cognitive mastery | |
| | Contemplation | Sustained openness to experience | |
| | Foreboding | Growing apprehension before deeper psychic contact | |

| *Domain of the Surrender Process* | *Experiential Configuration* | *Illustrative Clinical Process* | *Anatomical Function (Metaphor)* |
| --- | --- | --- | --- |
| Releasement: Transformational Reorganization (Level C) | | | |
| | Shift | Change in the individual's relationship to psychic life | Circulatory and Endocrine Systems |
| | Gratitude | Recognition of relational and existential dependency | |
| | Love | Openness toward self and others | |
| | Wisdom | Experiential understanding emerging from lived encounter | |
| | Revealing | Previously hidden aspects of self becoming visible | |
| | Unconcealment | Continued unfolding of psychic truth | |
| | Dynamic Flow | Increased flexibility of psychic movement | |
| | Repetition | Re-encountering earlier experiential configurations with new capacities | |
| Limit Condition of Surrender (Level D) | | | |
| | A Nameless Dread | Encounter with unformulated emotional experience prior to symbolization | Limits of Containment / Breakdown of Internal Organization |

quiet, nonlinear rhythms of analytic work—where patients showed me what had to be in place before they could truly let go.

This book offers a map of surrender's internal anatomy: a living system that expands and contracts in response to meaning, contact, and safety. Some parts stabilize, others transform; some remain hidden for years. Each chapter explores a different structure within this system—tracing how surrender unfolds, where it gets blocked, and what makes emotional movement possible.

Although not represented as a discrete configuration, aggression exerts pressure throughout the model. Each capacity is tested by the patient's ability to tolerate ambivalence toward the object—longing and hostility intertwined. Dependency invites resentment; frustration tolerance invites anger; love presumes the survival of the object under attack. Without this integration, surrender risks collapsing into compliance rather than deepening into recognition.

Like the lungs filling without command, surrender is a function of being alive—not something we choose, but something we can learn to notice.

At certain thresholds in the model—particularly between Releasement levels—brief neurobiological reflections are included to complement the psychological and symbolic terrain. These are not intended to reduce psychic experience to brain function, but to reflect the inseparability of mind and body. Where the psyche loosens, the nervous system responds. Affect, pattern, and meaning are not only mental events—they are physiological processes, experienced through shifts in arousal, co-regulation, and emotional rhythm. These references offer another layer of understanding: a parallel anatomy in which surrender becomes not only thinkable, but livable.

## Note

1 Albert Einstein, *The World as I See It* (New York: Philosophical Library, 1949).

# 1 The Atmosphere of Surrender

## Containment, Transference, and the Therapeutic Field

Surrender is a word that often conjures images of defeat or submission, yet in psychoanalysis, it holds a deeper, more transformative meaning. It is a function of psychic anatomy—an involuntary system we can learn to recognize and respond to, even if we cannot entirely control it. At its core, surrender is about allowing oneself to engage fully with internal experiences, letting go of rigid defenses, and opening up to the possibility of change. This concept lies at the heart of psychoanalytic work, where both therapist and patient embark on a journey toward understanding and connection. For the patient, surrender is not a passive act but an active choice to encounter vulnerability and embrace the unknown.

Before outlining the formal configurations within the surrender model, it's essential to begin with the analytic atmosphere in which surrender first takes root. This is not yet the model, but the felt texture beneath it—the emotional and relational climate in which something begins to stir long before it is named.

### Transference, Countertransference, and the Shared Dream

One of the essential components of the therapeutic process is transference, the projection of the patient's feelings, expectations, and fears onto the therapist. This dynamic, though complex, is invaluable in the work of surrender, as it allows patients to explore hidden parts of themselves within the safety of the therapeutic relationship. Antonino Ferro refers to the therapeutic encounter as a kind of "shared dream," a collaborative narrative where patient and therapist engage in a co-created space that reveals unprocessed emotions and experiences.

In these moments of shared reverie, the therapist is not merely an observer but an active participant in the unfolding narrative. The therapist's own internal responses, known as countertransference, reveal hidden dynamics and allow aspects of the patient's inner world to be reflected and understood. For many patients, surrendering to this shared dream feels foreign, even frightening. It asks them to let down their guard and trust that this new kind of connection will not harm or overwhelm them.

DOI: 10.4324/9781003795803-2

## Containment and the Skin Ego

Surrender rarely emerges in the absence of containment. It requires an analytic atmosphere capable of receiving what the patient cannot yet bear alone. Within such a holding environment, to use Donald Winnicott's formulation, emotional experience can begin to unfold without immediate retreat into defense. The patient may gradually feel psychologically held in the work itself, much as the infant is held within the reliability of early caregiving. Without this containing field, surrender can feel dangerous, as though the patient's internal world might spill beyond what can be endured.

Didier Anzieu's concept of the *skin ego* captures this dimension of containment. Anzieu described it as a psychological boundary that holds emotional experience much as the skin holds the body. For some patients, this containing function was insufficiently established in early life, leaving the self exposed and permeable. In analytic work with such patients, the task often becomes the gradual establishment of an external holding environment sturdy enough for an internal sense of psychic 'skin' to begin forming.

## Differentiating Surrender from Submission and Masochism

To understand surrender within the therapeutic context, it is important to distinguish it from concepts such as submission and masochism, which are often mistakenly conflated with it. In his seminal paper "Masochism, Submission, and Surrender" (1990), Emmanuel Ghent provides an important framework for making this distinction. Ghent proposed that surrender is a liberating movement in which defensive control is relinquished so that experience can be encountered more authentically. Unlike submission or masochism, which organize the self around compliance, suffering, or the appeasement of external authority, surrender preserves agency while allowing the person to encounter previously defended aspects of the self.

As Emmanuel Ghent (1990) wrote,

> Submission entails compliance in the service of adaptation to an external power or internalized ideal... Surrender, by contrast, refers to the letting down of defensive barriers that previously had kept one hidden from oneself and thereby precluded the possibility of genuine closeness with another.
>
> (p. 108)

This distinction is central to the therapeutic work that follows, where surrender becomes a pathway for accessing deeper and more authentic aspects of the self, not a sacrifice of agency but a reclaiming of it.

## Early Currents: What Surrender Begins to Feel Like

In the earliest phases of therapy, I'm not looking for breakthroughs or insights. I'm listening for texture—moments when something shifts just slightly in the field. A pause. A change in tone. A stray word that wasn't carefully managed.

Sometimes it shows up in a patient like Winston, who arrives dishevelled, self-deprecating, and avoids eye contact. He's not consciously seeking help—he's testing the space, often by creating a kind of chaos around him to see if I'll flinch. His surrender, if it comes, won't be verbal. It will be in the moment he doesn't apologize for existing.

Or it appears in someone like Gabriella, who speaks crisply and kindly and avoids needing anything at all. Then one day she says, almost in passing, "I nearly didn't come today."

She doesn't elaborate. The comment sits there, slightly out of place. I don't follow it immediately. I listen for what has made its way into the room that she hasn't quite taken back.

These are not stages. They are signals—subtle shifts in the field that suggest the patient has begun, in some fragile way, to imagine letting go.

## Embracing Dependency and Trust

One of the paradoxes of surrender is that it requires dependency, a concept many patients experience as uncomfortable or even shameful. In contemporary culture, independence and autonomy are often prized to such a degree that dependency comes to be equated with weakness. Within the therapeutic relationship, however, the capacity to depend on another person, the therapist, can represent a psychologically significant shift.

André Green's concept of the "Dead Mother Complex" speaks to what happens when early caregiving is emotionally absent or withdrawn. In such cases, dependency doesn't feel difficult—it feels dangerous. Gabriella, a retired schoolteacher in her 60s, learned early that expressing a need could shift something in the room—often not in her favor. Her mother could turn sharply when demands were made; her father's presence rarely extended beyond the surface. She adapted by relying on herself, keeping her needs contained. Over time, the analytic work pressed gently against that solitude, not through confrontation but through consistency. She once said, "I hate that I need this," then returned the next week, early, and sat for the full session without speaking.

Winston, a physician from a long-established Boston family, presented differently. His life was marked by acts of chaotic generosity—letting unstable people live in his home, neglecting his own care. He did not present with a clear wish to be held. Instead, he brought situations into the room that strained the possibility of it. The therapeutic frame had to remain consistent before he could begin to register it as something reliable.

In both cases, surrender was not a moment of collapse, but a gradual shift in what could be tolerated—dependence, contact, the presence of another.

## Trusting the Process

Trust doesn't begin with certainty—it begins with risk. And in therapy, that risk often takes the form of staying in the room when every part of the psyche wants to bolt.

Trusting the process means recognizing that surrender is not a straight path. The psyche may pause, circle back, or go still for long stretches. This doesn't mean nothing is happening. Often, what appears to be stalling reflects a form of psychic digestion, as internal systems prepare themselves to move again.

Even when there are no visible signs of progress—or when regression appears to dominate—the unconscious continues its work beneath awareness. Something is always being metabolized, reorganized, or protected. This invisible movement is often outside the conscious reach of both patient and therapist. It persists even in silence, even when sessions feel disconnected, and even when the two are not meeting at all.

In the early phases of the surrender process, particularly as dependency begins to emerge, patients often experience themselves as lagging behind—aware of what is possible, yet unable to move toward it. The pressure to advance can itself become a defense, narrowing the field rather than opening it. What is required instead is the capacity to remain in contact with that tension without resolving it prematurely, allowing something to take shape that cannot be forced.

Sometimes trust appears in a simple form: not knowing, and remaining, nonetheless.

## What Can't Be Thought Until It Is Re-Experienced

Without some degree of regression, much of this work stalls. True surrender often requires a soft undoing of the 'adult self'—the one who manages, performs, and stays in control. In its place, something less formed begins to emerge: a younger state, or a more primitive need, or even just a murmur of emotion that never had language.

If this regression is met with anxiety, silence, or interpretation too soon, the patient retreats. But when it is met with steady presence and allowed to remain where it is, something begins to open.

One patient once described it as "not knowing what age I am when I talk to you." She then quickly changed the subject. It was not yet something that could be approached directly, but the door had opened.

These are the moments that matter—not because they resolve anything, but because they signal that something deeper has begun to stir.

If these unthought experiences return not simply as memory, but as affective weather in the analytic room, then both patient and therapist are changed by their emergence. But what the therapist can allow—and what the therapist must hold—are not the same. Before turning to the surrender process itself, it's important to consider the ethical position of the therapist within this dynamic.

## Ethics and the Limits of Surrender in the Therapeutic Dyad

Although surrender is explored throughout this book as a process that unfolds in both therapist and patient, it must be emphasized that the therapist's surrender is of a different order—bounded, partial, and always in service of the patient's unfolding. The therapist cannot, and should not, surrender in the same way. The analytic task requires holding in mind both the reverberations of one's own internal process and the ethical responsibility to remain available, receptive, and protective of the analytic frame.

In this model, surrender is not an act but an internal orientation—an openness to what is not yet known, a loosening of certainty, a capacity to allow feeling to move before it becomes formulated. The therapist may find themselves drawn into states of reverie, emotional immersion, or disorientation, but must simultaneously retain the ability to reflect on these states rather than be absorbed by them. This is a paradoxical stance—like a surfer riding a wave while staying attuned to the shore. The therapist must remain open to being moved, while still able to think.

This capacity to surrender within the analytic function depends not only on the therapist's internal stance but also on the patient's capacity to permit such openness. When the patient remains defensive, overly intellectualized, or fixed on interrogating the therapist, the shared analytic field narrows. The therapist's reverie, in these moments, may be dulled or distorted. Surrender in the therapist is not enacted in a vacuum—it depends on the patient's willingness to risk internal contact.

Critically, the therapist must also remain alert to their own unconscious gratifications. Unacknowledged narcissistic seductions—especially when colluded with by the patient—undermine the surrender process entirely. What may appear as mutuality can in fact be a reenactment of submission and control, in which the patient becomes a vehicle for the therapist's unmet needs. Such moments, however subtle, may resemble surrender but are instead a form of enactment, often intense but ethically ruptured. True surrender cannot occur where the ethical asymmetry of the analytic relationship is denied or blurred.

In this sense, the therapist's surrender must always include the capacity to stop. To step back. To think. It is not the loss of self, but the expansion of internal space through which another may begin to emerge. The deepest form of surrender the therapist can offer is the refusal to act on unconscious desire—remaining instead in that difficult, generative space between contact and control.

This ethical framing is deepened by Jessica Benjamin's work on mutual recognition and Thirdness, which expands the scope of surrender from an internal act to an intersubjective achievement. For Benjamin (2018), the aim of therapy is not merely individual insight but the emergence of an intersubjective space where each mind can register the other without erasing difference. Recognition is not the product of fusion, nor is it possible within defended separateness; it arises in the tension between connectedness and differentiation. This tension is inherently asymmetrical in therapy. The therapist bears a greater responsibility—not only to remain receptive, but to metabolize what the patient cannot yet hold. Their surrender must be partial and consciously held, not enacted for its own release, but in service of what the patient is struggling to bring into being.

This book has therefore separated the patient's surrender from the therapist's—not to deny their mutual influence, but to respect the ethical and developmental complexity of their convergence. Surrender, at its depth, is not for merger or withdrawal, but for recognition: a state in which the self remains distinct and yet allows itself to be known. Recognition, then, is not an outcome of surrender but its ethical horizon.

# 2 Civilization's Pursuit of Surrender

Our lives are bookended by surrender—in birth and in death. In between, many people spend their entire lives attempting to avoid surrender, driven by a desire to control and contain their experience of life. The concept of surrender has appeared across disciplines, from meditation and yoga to art and psychoanalysis, each seeking to understand and harness the power of letting go. But true surrender, especially in the therapeutic sense, requires a profound engagement with vulnerability, one that exposes us to the possibility of transformation and, in some cases, healing.

Civilization itself —particularly in its modern Western form—seems to hold an ambivalent stance toward surrender, valuing autonomy, control, and independence while often viewing vulnerability as a weakness. Literature, philosophy, and religion have grappled with this tension for centuries. In F. Scott Fitzgerald's *The Great Gatsby*, for example, Jay Gatsby's refusal to let go of his dream of reclaiming the past leads to his downfall. His inability to surrender to reality and accept the limits of his control reflects a broader societal resistance to letting go. Conversely, in Tolstoy's *Anna Karenina*, Anna's pursuit of romantic surrender defies societal norms, exposing her to both the liberation of following her desires and the tragic consequences of breaking free from imposed constraints.

In psychoanalysis, surrender is often less dramatic than in literature, though no less transformative. While psychoanalysis has long explored the capacities that make transformation possible—dependence, frustration tolerance, regression, symbolization, and the integration of ambivalence—it has rarely organized these capacities explicitly around the phenomenon of surrender. The model that follows does not introduce new psychic functions; rather, it brings familiar ones into structural relationship, tracing how they build upon one another to form a developmental sequence within analytic work. What appears mystical at the far edge of experience is, in fact, made possible by the gradual strengthening of psychic structure.

As the chapters progress, we will see how surrender unfolds through these interrelated capacities, each demanding a deeper level of openness, vulnerability, and trust. The individuals in this book—Winston, Bill, Jerome, Tinsley, and Gabriella—illuminate different aspects of this process as they

DOI: 10.4324/9781003795803-3

encounter its configurations in distinct and personal ways. Through them, the model moves from outline to encounter, from theoretical sequence into lived experience.

The five clinical figures who recur throughout the book represent different psychological organizations, each encountering surrender from a distinct defensive position.

Yet even before surrender becomes livable, something in the individual must be willing to risk exposure. Some people learn early that expressing need is unsafe, even dangerous. They develop a vigilant stance toward vulnerability, protecting themselves through emotional restraint or withdrawal. These defenses are often invisible to others—but within, they make surrender feel intolerable. Therapy may become the first place where the body is no longer under surveillance, where hunger—for recognition, for contact—can finally be acknowledged. To understand surrender, we must first recognize what makes it so difficult: a culture that equates control with strength, and histories that teach us to hide our longing.

In her translation of *Dark Night of the Soul*, Mirabai Starr (2002) captures the essence of surrender as a journey into unknowing:

> I entered into unknowing
> and remained there,
> knowing nothing.
> This place transcends all thought…
> …I discovered the science
> of perfect peace, perfect holiness!
> A direct path opened
> through the heart of solitude.
> This journey transcends all thought.
> (Starr, 2002, p. 89)

Starr's rendering of St. John of the Cross captures the phenomenon of surrender at its most profound—a radical unknowing that this model identifies as *A Nameless Dread*, the furthest reach of therapeutic surrender within analytic work. It is a psychic state in which familiar structures of self and meaning loosen, allowing contact with what had previously remained unformulated. This is not a permanent dissolution, nor does it unfold identically for every patient. For some, it appears primarily as sustained contact with psychic material that cannot yet be symbolized; for others, it may involve a more destabilizing loosening of previously consolidated identity structures. What defines this configuration is not annihilation or transcendence, but the capacity to remain present at the edge of psychic unformulation without retreat.

The configurations presented in this model—from the early foundations of the *Closed* state, *Capacity to Depend, Open-Ended Attention*, and *Capacity to Regress*, to the deeper relational capacities that follow—build an inner structure that makes such surrender livable. These early capacities are not mystical in themselves, but they are essential for cultivating the psychic stability required to enter the destabilizing, transformative experiences that arise in the later capacities—*Ecstasy, Foreboding, Shift,* and ultimately, *A Nameless Dread.* Without this preparatory work, the psyche cannot endure the depth of transformation these capacities invite. The presence of another mind—especially one that can remain receptive without intrusion—makes this level of surrender not only possible, but survivable.

This chapter situates surrender within a broader cultural and psychological tension—between control and vulnerability, autonomy and exposure. What follows shifts from that frame to the internal architecture that makes surrender possible within analytic work. The configurations ahead trace how psychic capacities are built, consolidated, and tested, revealing surrender not as a single dramatic gesture, but as a developmental achievement that unfolds over time.

# Part I

# Foundational Capacities

## The Organs of Psychic Survival

Surrender does not emerge in the absence of psychic stability. The foundational configurations are not transformative in themselves; they establish the conditions under which transformation may become tolerable. Like the autonomic functions of the heart, lungs, and skin, these capacities operate silently—until they fail. Their disruption is often more visible than their presence.

The configurations included here—the *Closed* state, *Capacity to Depend, Open-Ended Attention*, and *Capacity to Regress*—can be understood as the organs of psychic survival. They support rudimentary affect regulation, enable nascent trust, and make possible a provisional contact with experience without collapse. Esther Bick's concept of the psychic skin is particularly resonant here: just as the infant relies on the containing function of the mother to hold together a fragile sense of self, these early capacities provide a kind of internal envelope that preserves coherence in the face of emotional intensity.

Their function is not insight, but stabilization. They protect against disintegration and preserve the psychic viability within which surrender may become tolerable, or even conceivable. The chapters that follow explore the conditions associated with this structural groundwork—conditions in which surrender may appear, not as an act of will, but as a readiness supported from within.

Neurobiologically, the foundational configurations within the surrender model correspond to systems involved in safety, attachment, and affect regulation. At this level, the psyche is organized less by symbolic processing and more by autonomic responses—particularly those associated with brainstem activity, vagal regulation, and right hemisphere attachment processes. Co-regulation with the therapist may contribute to the stabilization of threat-based responses, making different forms of contact more available within the analytic setting. This work is associated with the emergence of conditions in which symbolic containment, reflective function, and

DOI: 10.4324/9781003795803-4

transformation may become possible—not as outcomes that follow, but as capacities that can be supported under certain internal and relational conditions.

The *Closed* state can be understood as a defensive configuration that protects psychic survival through withdrawal, constriction, or refusal.

# 3 Closed

Surrender is often first encountered as resistance. For many, even momentary letting go can feel deeply unsettling. This configuration, which I term the *Closed* state, is where patients encounter their strongest defenses, standing guard over the parts of themselves they dare not expose. In the therapeutic setting, this resistance manifests as an inability to connect with one's deeper emotions, an instinctive closing off from vulnerability. For some patients, movement beyond this defensive position may take years of analytic work, and in certain cases it may never fully occur.

## The Challenge of Moving Beyond the Closed State

Not all patients are able to move beyond the *Closed* state. For some, the prospect of loosening control, even incrementally, feels overwhelming. The idea of depending on another person, even within the safe boundaries of the therapeutic relationship, can be so unsettling that these individuals may choose to withdraw from therapy rather than face that vulnerability. Patients in the *Closed* state often feel that their defenses are necessary for survival, and the idea of surrendering any of them can provoke intense fear or resistance. In these cases, therapy may end prematurely, with the patient unable or unwilling to progress toward deeper surrender.

The configurations within the surrender model do not unfold linearly. Movement beyond the *Closed* state does not preclude its return; under certain conditions, familiar defenses reassert themselves. What appears as regression reflects a shift in what can be borne. Earlier configurations reappear under altered internal conditions, especially when they are faced with deeper aspects of surrender. This fluctuation reflects the complexity of human psychology and the layered nature of surrender, where growth is not a straight line but a journey with twists, turns, and occasional returns to old patterns.

## The *Closed* State: A Fortress of Defenses

In the *Closed* state, patients operate under an imperative to control, often relying on intellectualization, pride, and an insatiable need for rational

DOI: 10.4324/9781003795803-5

explanations. In the clinical material that informed the original surrender model, three defensive tendencies repeatedly appeared within this closed position: *self-will*, the drive to maintain control over emotional processes and outcomes even at the expense of deeper understanding; *calculating*, a tendency to intellectualize or rationalize emotions while avoiding the raw experience of feeling; and *pride*, a refusal to allow vulnerability that keeps emotional defenses firmly in place.

Individuals in the *Closed* state are often over-reliant on these defenses, which serve to protect them from the perceived threat of losing control. They may experience moments of intense self-criticism or persecutory thoughts, reinforcing the belief that surrender is psychologically unsafe. Beneath this position lies a fundamental reluctance to trust—both in the therapist and in themselves. In this state, patients may demand answers to the 'why' behind every feeling, expecting a logical explanation that can be dissected and controlled.

This control, however, comes at a cost. By clinging to self-will and pride, they limit their ability to experience emotions directly, creating an emotional distance that restricts deeper psychological movement.

## The Struggle to Surrender

In this *Closed* state, surrender feels counterintuitive. Our society, with its emphasis on autonomy, strength, and certainty, primes individuals to avoid vulnerability. We are taught to equate control with safety and independence with self-worth. In therapy, this cultural conditioning translates to a hesitation to let go, an instinct to rationalize and compartmentalize emotions rather than experience them directly. Letting go of control, even momentarily, feels like an admission of defeat.

But surrender, as we shall see, is not about defeat. It is a process of discovery—of uncovering aspects of the self that have long been hidden. Yet to the closed mind, surrender feels alien, as if opening oneself to vulnerability would lead to disintegration. This fear often keeps patients locked within their defenses, unable to move forward in their therapeutic journey.

### *Tinsley*

Tinsley, a thirty-something self-branded 'Creative Consultant' with a carefully honed aesthetic and a trail of abruptly ended therapies, entered the room the way one might enter a gallery—knowing the light would hit her just right. She spoke fluently, even fluently about pain, but the words were lacquered, well-arranged, the kind that invited admiration rather than inquiry. Her voice always had a certain crispness to it, like she was speaking into a podcast mic just out of frame.

The stories she brought were curated. A break-up, rebranded as growth. A betrayal, recast as discernment. Her emotions didn't arrive raw; they arrived post-produced. When she said, "I've already processed it," it felt less like a claim and more like a pre-emptive defense—against what might surface if we slowed down.

She once described a friend cutting her off abruptly. "It showed me who she really was," she said, with the practiced certainty of someone who'd posted it as a caption. She paused, as if waiting for me to nod in agreement.

"What was the feeling before it became a conclusion?" I asked.

There was a blink. A flicker. Then the room reassembled.

"I mean—what's the point? I've already moved on."

The space filled with the weight of something ungrieved. Not denied, exactly, just never unwrapped.

With Tinsley, it wasn't what she said that told the story—it was the speed of the pivot, the way the affect vanished just before landing. There was always a kind of management happening. She didn't defend against emotion by overthinking it—she defended by making it beautiful.

She had been coming for a couple of years, consistently. Always punctual, always composed, rarely off-script. The field between us often felt like a polished floor: reflective, sleek, and difficult to grip. Moments of warmth or softness threatened to cloud the shine.

Now and then, I would notice a faint tightness around her mouth when I asked a question she hadn't rehearsed an answer for. If I lingered too long in a silence, her posture would subtly sharpen. It wasn't hostility—it was adjustment. I was being edited. She never accused, never objected. She simply smoothed the surface back over.

There were patterns: slight shifts in tone, a glance just past me, a pivot in topic. It was like watching a security system respond to a perceived breach. Something inside her was scanning—sorting the safe from the unsafe, the useful from the intrusive.

What she couldn't hold inside, she arranged outside.

And still, something in her kept showing up.

### *Bill*

Bill, a former military technician in his late 50s whose quiet resignation had begun to calcify into emotional flatness, entered therapy like someone clocking in to a shift—punctual, polite, and completely unreachable. He sat still, hands folded, face unreadable. The air around him felt compressed, like a room that hadn't been aired in years. He didn't resist therapy, but he didn't inhabit it either. He was present the way a chair is present.

When I asked why he'd come, he said, "My wife's tired of talking to herself."

He didn't offer more. He rarely did. When I asked about his childhood, he recited data—number of siblings, the year his father died. But nothing had texture. Nothing had mood. "No point going backwards," he said. "It's done."

His inner world felt like a garage with the lights off. Not empty, but not in use.

One day, he mentioned walking in on his wife crying in the kitchen.

"I didn't ask what was wrong," he said. "I just emptied the dishwasher."

I asked what stopped him.

He blinked, then looked away. "I guess I didn't want to make it worse. Or hear something I couldn't fix."

There was a long silence. Not charged. Not tense. Just there.

"I used to be good at things," he said. "I knew what to do."

The sadness didn't show in his tone. It showed in the way he didn't lift his eyes.

The field with Bill often felt like fog—not because things were unclear, but because they were so thinly expressed. Emotion leaked at the edges but never pooled. He didn't shut things down dramatically—he just never opened the door.

He wasn't yet surrendering. But he was starting to hear the echo of his own quiet. The defenses weren't cracking, but he was beginning to wonder what was on the other side of them. That wondering, barely spoken, was the beginning of something.

## What It Asks of the Therapist

Working with a patient in the *Closed* state can stir up a unique kind of countertransference: not resistance, but invisibility. The therapist may feel erased, irrelevant, or inert—like the session is happening in a vacuum. There may be a pull to work harder, to interpret prematurely, or to emotionally 'perform' in the hope of cracking something open.

But the *Closed* state does not yield to pressure. It responds only to the therapist's capacity to stay present without demand. This requires a quiet kind of faith: that the work is happening beneath the surface, even when nothing seems to be moving.

With Bill, it was the steady emptiness that tested the frame. He didn't push the therapist out; he simply never let anyone in. The air felt thinned out, the contact minimal. He wasn't rejecting interpretation—he was bypassing the need for it altogether. The therapist's challenge was to resist filling the space or demanding entry, to recognize the defense not as absence, but as a lived strategy. What appeared as flatness was a structure built from endurance. The countertransference could feel like dullness, futility, or even quiet despair—not unlike what Bill had likely been defending against for decades.

With Tinsley, the defense was more stylized. Her self-curation left little room for spontaneity or rupture. Emotion arrived dressed and rehearsed, stylized into insight before it could threaten to overwhelm. Underneath the fluency, however, projection did its work. Moments of misattunement—or even subtle attunement—could provoke a shift in the transference: the therapist was suddenly too interested or not interested enough, intrusive or indifferent. The sense of being watched and evaluated was constant, as though any wrong note might confirm an internal certainty that the other would exploit, diminish, or fail her. The therapist had to feel the tension of that scrutiny without retreating into defensiveness or self-doubt.

In both cases, the defenses served to organize experience in the face of something unrepresentable. The therapist must be able to tolerate being misperceived—felt as a persecutory or absent figure—and still remain in contact. Not neutral in the blank sense, but steady: neither withdrawing from the affect nor rushing to resolve it.

At times, the therapist may experience self-doubt, boredom, or helplessness—feelings that mirror what the patient is defending against. The task is to stay with these internal states without acting them out, and without demanding reciprocity. The *Closed* state asks the therapist to sustain an atmosphere in which thinking can be born, not imposed. Interpretation too soon may feel like intrusion; waiting too long can become collusion. The work lies in inhabiting the tension.

When what Thomas Ogden called the analytic third begins to take shape—a shared psychological space co-created by patient and therapist, distinct from either alone—it marks a shift from parallel monologues to a jointly held experience (Ogden, 1994). In this space, meanings begin to constellate not through direct insight, but through mutual presence and reverie. The therapist's task is not to extract content from the patient but to join them in enduring the psychic atmosphere together, until what was unspeakable begins to find its contour. It is an act not of decoding, but of dwelling-with. In some treatments, that co-presence may take years to be felt. But it begins here.

## The Cost of Staying Closed

*Closed* doesn't always look the same. Sometimes it's a brand. Sometimes it's silence. Tinsley polished her surfaces until they gleamed; Bill let the dust settle around him undisturbed. One performed herself into containment. The other disappeared into routine.

In both rooms, something remained untouched. Not because it wasn't there, but because neither of them could risk what might follow if it surfaced unfiltered. For Tinsley, letting go of control meant risking unraveling. For Bill, turning toward feeling meant awakening something long buried—something that might no longer have a place to go.

The *Closed* state doesn't shout. It doesn't storm out. It sits quietly at the edge of the session, whispering that nothing needs to change. That it's better not to look.

But over time, the cost of staying closed accrues—measured not in crisis, but in dimming. In what never gets spoken. In what never has a witness.

## Toward Surrender

It wouldn't look dramatic. Not a confession or a breakdown. It would look like hesitation held just a second longer. A sentence that doesn't finish itself.

A gaze that lingers instead of shifting away. The performance pausing. The silence being allowed to echo.

Surrender, here, begins when the impulse to tidy or disappear is delayed—just long enough for something raw, unframed, and not yet named to make contact.

In the chapters that follow, we explore how the process of surrender unfolds across its configurations. Each introduces a different demand on the patient's relation to control, challenging the structures that sustain resistance. But it begins here, in the *Closed* state, where the walls are high and the defenses are fierce. What is required is not breakthrough, but the first loosening of those defenses—making possible a deeper experience of the self and a more immediate contact with life.

# 4 The Capacity to Depend

As the defenses of the *Closed* state begin to soften, a new and more complex demand emerges: the *Capacity to Depend*. This capacity is essential for deepening the work, as it involves a willingness to trust another and to rely on them. In therapy, this means surrendering to the therapeutic relationship itself—a process that can provoke intense fear in those who have learned to equate dependency with vulnerability or weakness.

## The Struggle with Dependency

In many Western cultures, independence is highly prized, while dependency is often viewed as a weakness. This cultural conditioning can make it especially difficult for individuals to embrace healthy forms of dependency—even in relationships where trust is foundational, such as therapy. For many patients, admitting a need for another person evokes shame, as if they are regressing into helplessness. But therapeutic dependency is not about relinquishing autonomy. Rather, it is about developing a secure base from which one can safely explore deeper, often hidden, parts of the self.

Winnicott's concept of the "holding environment" (1965) is particularly relevant in this context. In early childhood, a nurturing caregiver provides an environment where the child feels safe to explore and grow. This secure base fosters a sense of trust, allowing the child to experience emotions without overwhelming fear. In therapy, the therapist recreates this holding environment, providing a space where the patient can begin to depend on them, opening themselves to emotions and experiences that might otherwise feel too threatening.

## The Influence of Early Attachment

Attachment theory, first articulated by John Bowlby (1969, 1973), draws attention to the enduring influence of early relationships with caregivers on the individual's capacity to trust and depend on others. Where early attachment relationships were experienced as stable and responsive, the individual may later tolerate forms of dependency without excessive

DOI: 10.4324/9781003795803-6

anxiety. When early care was marked by neglect, inconsistency, or emotional unavailability, dependency can instead evoke fears of abandonment, intrusion, or loss of self. These early relational configurations do not remain confined to childhood; they tend to reappear in later relationships, often becoming especially visible in the patient's capacity—or difficulty—in relying on the therapist.

For some patients, particularly those who have suffered early relational failures, dependency in therapy can feel especially risky. André Green's "Dead Mother Complex" (1983/1993) describes a situation in which an emotionally absent caregiver leaves the child with a pervasive sense of emptiness, complicating the capacity for later relationships. Patients who have endured this form of relational absence may find it nearly impossible to trust another person deeply. The fear of repeating this abandonment can lead to self-sufficiency or defensive detachment, even when they consciously long for connection.

## Gabriella

Gabriella, a retired schoolteacher with a careful voice and a face that held everything close, arrived in therapy like someone stepping into a room she half-expected not to exist. At the start of each session, she glanced around, as if confirming that everything was still in place. Her presence carried an unspoken rule—that to lean might break something.

Words came slowly. She spoke of routines and neighbors, of how the world had gotten louder. Beneath it was a kind of stillness—not restful, but held in place.

In one session, she described a dream: a child waiting outside a door that never opened, though the light inside stayed on. "She knew it wasn't her place," Gabriella said. She offered it without affect. But the dream didn't need interpreting—it was the room. The child, the door, the waiting—already present between us.

At times, she watched me closely, as if gauging whether I would remain. Her voice stayed even. Her words were measured. But something in the room felt held under tension.

I said, "Maybe part of what makes this so hard is how long you've waited without knocking."

She looked down. After a pause: "I don't want to need you… but I think I do."

Nothing dramatic followed. But something in the structure shifted.

In the weeks that followed, she began to test the space. She mentioned a dream and asked what I thought. She referred to a previous session, then moved away from it. Once, she said, "I guess I missed this," and did not elaborate.

These movements were small. She would approach, then pull back. Ask, then seem unsure she had asked. Her transference did not press forward. It gathered slowly—in the pacing, in what was returned to, in what was not withdrawn.

Dependency did not arrive as something spoken. It formed in the space between sessions—in her returning, in what she allowed to remain. I did not name it. I stayed with it. And over time, something in the room became possible that had not been before.

## Winston

Winston had never described himself as someone who needed people. In his words, he was the one others relied on—friends needing a place to stay, former colleagues calling in favors, people passing through who somehow remained. His house was rarely empty.

Early in therapy, he spoke about this as if it were incidental. "I don't like seeing people stuck," he said, describing how a former neighbor had moved into his guest room. "I've got the space."

I asked what it was like, having people in his home all the time.

He shrugged. "Better than the alternative."

"What's the alternative?"

He paused. "I don't know. Just... too much space, I guess."

In one session, after a difficult week, he arrived more withdrawn than usual. "They're driving me nuts," he said. "Left the stove on twice. I almost lost it."

"And they're still there."

"Yeah." He looked down. "Kicked everyone out once. Place was empty for a couple days."

"What was that like?"

He shifted in his seat. "Didn't like it."

He didn't elaborate.

Over time, a pattern began to take shape. Winston did not speak about needing anyone. But he filled his space in ways that made absence difficult to encounter. When the house emptied, he brought someone back.

In one session, he mentioned, almost in passing, "Sometimes I leave things broken. Not big things. Just... stuff I could fix."

I waited.

"So someone has to come by," he added. "Take a look."

We let that sit.

He gave a brief, uneven smile. "I don't know. It's stupid."

Nothing was resolved. But something had come into view—not as a conclusion, but as a possibility he had not fully turned away from.

## What It Asks of the Therapist

In the earliest stirrings of dependency, the therapist may feel subtle pressure: toward softening, over-functioning, or disengaging. These movements in the countertransference are rarely overt. More often, they reflect the patient's ambivalence—approaching need without fully allowing it.

With Gabriella, the therapist may feel an impulse to lean in, to respond with particular care. Her measured presence, shaped by a long adaptation to not needing, can evoke a protective stance—an inclination to anticipate rupture and move carefully around it. But too much caution risks repeating what she already knows: that others adjust without fully meeting her. The task is to remain present without withdrawing or over-modulating—to hold contact without diluting it. The countertransference may carry a sense of waiting, which must be tolerated without pressing it into expression.

With Winston, the pressure shifts. The therapist may feel drawn to intervene, to organize, to relieve. His pattern of filling his life with others can pull the therapist into a familiar position—responding to what is visible while missing what is absent. His needs are not directly stated; they emerge through the situations he creates. The countertransference may move between frustration and a pull to provide what he does not ask for. To maintain the frame here requires restraint—to not repair too quickly, and to allow what is avoided to begin to register.

Across both cases, dependency does not appear directly. It emerges in small moments—in hesitation, in return, in what is left unfinished. The therapist may feel the urge to interpret or reassure, but this capacity requires something more contained. The work is to notice what is beginning and to remain steady as it takes shape.

Countertransference in this phase is less about reaction than about tolerance: the ability to register a patient's need without moving to meet or reject it prematurely. Dependency is not yet stable enough to be named. It is a tentative movement toward contact, and it must be held as such.

## Transforming Relationships Through Dependency

From a Winnicottian perspective, dependency in the therapeutic relationship reactivates early needs for a caregiver capable of holding—of providing emotional attunement without intrusion or withdrawal (Winnicott, 1960). At times, this may take on a quality reminiscent of the child's search in *Are You My Mother?*—an unformulated longing for a reliable presence that was absent or inconsistent.

In the analytic setting, this longing often emerges as an idealization of the therapist. Winnicott cautioned against interpreting such states too quickly, emphasizing instead the necessity of allowing dependency to unfold within a holding environment. What matters is not the resolution of dependency, but the therapist's capacity to endure it without withdrawal or retaliation.

Within this sustained presence, something begins to shift. The patient encounters the therapist not only as needed, but as separate—capable of being relied upon, but also of frustrating, failing, and even being hated. The capacity to remain in relationship under these conditions marks a crucial movement in the surrender process. Dependency is no longer organized around merger or avoidance, but becomes the ground from which a more reciprocal, reality-based form of relatedness can emerge.

## Justification for the Placement of this Capacity

The *Capacity to Depend* is foundational for what follows. Without it, the later capacities cannot be sustained. As reliance on the therapist becomes possible, patients begin to approach their experience differently—less organized around control, more able to remain in contact with what emerges. The therapist's steadiness makes this contact bearable.

As Antonino Ferro notes, each therapeutic encounter is a journey into the unknown. The therapist and patient navigate this journey together, venturing into uncharted territories of the psyche. For the patient, surrendering to dependency enables a richer engagement with this journey, as they come to trust that the therapist will guide and support them through the complexities that arise.

## Concluding Reflections

The *Capacity to Depend* marks a decisive shift in the therapeutic process. What once felt dangerous—turning toward another in need—becomes possible, though rarely without conflict. Patients must confront the very experiences that taught them dependency could not be survived.

In Gabriella, dependency emerges as a gradual willingness to risk being met. In Winston, it appears more obliquely—disguised through care for others or embedded in chaotic relational patterns that keep his own needs at a distance. In both, the movement toward dependency is uneven, shaped by fear as much as longing.

What begins as a tentative reliance on the therapist can, over time, open into something more fundamental: the capacity to remain in relationship without collapsing into self-sufficiency or dissolving into need. In this way, dependency is not relinquished but transformed—becoming a condition through which deeper forms of contact and ultimately surrender, can occur.

From this ground, a further shift becomes possible: attention can begin to loosen from its defensive organization and turn more fully toward experience itself.

# 5 Open-Ended Attention

As patients engage the configurations of the surrender model, their mode of experiencing begins to shift. What emerges here is a form of attention that can be described as open-ended. This reflects a loosening of the rigid defenses of the *Closed* state and a movement beyond the tentative reliance associated with the *Capacity to Depend*. Attention becomes less organized around control, explanation, or categorization, and more able to remain with experience as it unfolds. Thoughts and emotions can be encountered without immediate judgment or the need for resolution.

In psychoanalytic therapy, this form of attention is essential. It allows both patient and therapist to remain present to the unfolding moment without prematurely imposing meaning. As this capacity develops, the patient begins to loosen the grip of rationalization and tolerate the ambiguity that accompanies deeper forms of self-experience and surrender.

The classical analytic invitation to free associate—to speak without premature censorship—appears simple, yet it often reveals the patient's central difficulty less through the content of what is said than through the precise ways spontaneous thought cannot proceed. Mind may tighten into explanation, collapse into blankness, seek relevance, or turn away at the threshold of feeling. Such impediments are not secondary obstacles to the work; they are among its clearest expressions. Open-ended attention creates the conditions in which these constraints can gradually be recognized and relinquished.

## The Concept of Open-Ended Attention

The idea of open-ended attention is rooted in the writings of thinkers such as Simone Weil (2009) and William James (1890/1950). Weil described attention as a spiritual and ethical practice, one that invites individuals to detach themselves from personal desires and become fully receptive to the truth and suffering of others. This receptive state goes beyond mere observation; it becomes a transformative force necessary for surrender, creating a space where genuine emotional work can unfold. William James, whose work laid the foundation for both modern psychology and pragmatist philosophy, saw

DOI: 10.4324/9781003795803-7

attention as an active force that organizes experience. "My experience is what I agree to attend to," he wrote (p. 402), pointing to how our inner life is shaped by what we choose—or are able—to notice. In therapy, this openness to experience captures the essence of therapeutic surrender—the ability to be open to what is, rather than clinging to fixed interpretations or assumptions. By maintaining an open-ended attention, patients can explore deeper parts of themselves without the compulsion to understand or explain every emotion.

## Jerome

Jerome, a highly successful attorney in his early 40s, had built his life around clarity, structure, and control. In court, every word mattered. Every detail was accounted for. This precision extended into his inner life—he approached therapy much like he approached litigation: with focus, discipline, and a subtle but ever-present defense against uncertainty.

Early in our work, Jerome struggled with the ambiguity inherent in open-ended attention. He was not overtly resistant—he wanted to understand himself—but he wanted to do so on his terms. When asked about his dreams, he often arrived with a carefully written summary, complete with speculative interpretations and bullet-pointed insights. "I've been thinking about this one all week," he would say, holding his notes. "I think the train represents my career, and the broken window might be a sign I'm avoiding something. Possibly intimacy."

What he couldn't yet tolerate was *not* knowing.

In one session, I asked Jerome to describe a recent dream aloud, slowly, without referring to his notes or offering any interpretation. At first, he complied, but the moment an image emerged—a foggy platform, a suitcase left behind—he slipped into analysis. "I think the suitcase is about—" he began.

I gently interrupted. "What's it like just to stay with the image? The platform. The fog. The suitcase. Without knowing yet."

He looked at me, unsettled. "Honestly? It feels… inefficient. Like we're wasting time."

This moment captured the core tension of the configuration. For Jerome, not analyzing felt irresponsible. Letting an image simply be without turning it into something useful—into evidence—was profoundly uncomfortable.

Over time, however, he began to sense the value in holding things lightly. As he allowed himself to speak more freely, without striving for conclusions, he noticed new layers in his associations: flickers of childhood memories, fleeting emotions, the way his body tensed at certain moments. "I kept thinking about the suitcase again," he said one week. "But this time, I remembered how I used to pack and repack my bag as a kid when my mom was late coming home from her shift. I thought if I was ready to leave, maybe she'd stay."

This wasn't a polished insight. It was vulnerable. It emerged not from effortful thinking, but from letting go of effort altogether.

Jerome's journey into open-ended attention wasn't linear. He would return often to old habits of control—especially when feeling exposed. But gradually, he came to trust that meaning didn't always need to be extracted. Sometimes it arrived when he stopped reaching for it. What began as a challenge to his sense of efficiency turned into something more intimate: an invitation to be with himself in a way he had never quite allowed before.

## Bill

Bill came to therapy with no particular goal. "Figured it couldn't hurt," he said on the first day, voice flat. "Wife says I'm distant. Maybe I am."

His sessions reflected this flatness. Long pauses. Short answers. Stories without color. The therapist noticed how quickly Bill diverted away from anything that seemed emotionally charged.

"Sounds like that was a hard moment," she once said after he described an old friend's betrayal.

Bill shrugged. "Nah, it's life."

In another session, he recounted a dream where he stood in a field staring at a fence, not knowing if he should climb it. "Did you feel anything in the dream?" the therapist asked.

"Can't remember," he replied. "It was just... a fence."

But the session shifted when the therapist changed tack. "Do you notice anything in your body as you talk about it?"

Bill frowned, then rubbed his chest absently. "Weird tightness. Like someone's sitting on me. Happens sometimes."

"Can we stay with that feeling for a moment? No need to explain it. Just notice it."

The minutes stretched, Bill fidgeting, then settling. "It gets heavier when I talk about the fence," he admitted. "Like I'll have to climb it but I don't want to."

"And if we don't climb it, just sit here—what happens?"

Bill blinked, voice quieter. "Not much. But... it's not as bad as I thought."

Over time, these somatic moments became anchors. Bill's resistance to emotional content softened when approached indirectly—through body awareness rather than probing questions. He didn't like digging into the past, but he could stay longer with sensations, with small moments of attention that didn't demand answers.

In a later session, after another pause, Bill said, "It's easier to be quiet here than it is at home. Not empty. Just... quiet."

The therapist smiled gently. "Maybe that's a kind of attention too. One that doesn't need to fix or figure out."

Bill nodded. "Yeah. Maybe."

## What It Asks of the Therapist

Jerome's difficulty with open-ended attention highlights what this configuration quietly demands of the therapist: the ability to remain present, emotionally available, and psychologically spacious, even when the patient resists not-knowing. For someone like Jerome—who clings to clarity, analysis, and control—the therapist becomes a kind of counterpoint: holding space for what cannot yet be understood, without pressing or retreating.

With Bill, open-ended attention encounters a different obstacle: the absence of obvious emotional content. His sessions drift into silence, mundane details, or bodily observations that seem unimportant but carry hidden meaning. The therapist's challenge is to resist the pull to 'wake up' the session artificially—to avoid pushing for emotion or insight where Bill's system can only tolerate quiet witnessing. In Bill's transference, the therapist risks becoming an indifferent observer or a rescuing figure who forces aliveness too quickly. The countertransference can reflect this: a sense of boredom, uselessness, or restlessness may arise, tempting the therapist to over-structure the work or prematurely interpret in order to feel effective.

This is no small task. Open-ended attention, as Bion (1967/2014) describes it, requires the therapist to approach each session with "no memory, no desire, no understanding." It means staying close to the patient's material—words, images, silences—without rushing toward meaning. In Jerome's case, this often meant resisting the pull to affirm or interpret prematurely, even when his insights were intelligent and tempting to build upon. With Bill, it often meant tolerating the flatness of the field, sensing where quiet presence could allow something imperceptible to emerge—whether in the body, in fleeting feelings, or in subtle shifts of tone.

And yet, the therapist is not immune to the field. There are days when this kind of attention becomes more difficult—when the therapist, too, is struggling. Strong feelings such as irritation, protectiveness, longing, or even aversion may arise from countertransference or from the therapist's own life. With Jerome, there may be admiration or competitiveness over his intellect; with Bill, there may be frustration over his apparent detachment, or an unconscious desire to 'fix' his deadened affect. The therapist may subtly align with the patient's defenses—pressing for clarity with Jerome, avoiding the quiet with Bill—or find themselves moving the session along for their own comfort rather than the patient's need.

Recognizing these moments is essential. The therapist must be able to reflect on their own mental state and its impact on the space. If open-ended attention is to be sustained, the therapist needs internal room not only for the patient's uncertainty, but also for their own. The therapeutic container holds both minds—and both minds must be tended to.

Ultimately, what Jerome needed, what Bill needed, and what many patients need in this configuration, is a therapist who can stay with them in the fog of the unknown, without judgment or haste.

This means not just technical skill, but a kind of emotional sturdiness: the willingness to be with a patient who cannot yet surrender, without demanding that they do so. And when the therapist's own capacity falters, what is asked is not perfection, but awareness—a readiness to pause, reflect, and return again to the open space between knowing and not knowing.

## Justification of Placement

*Open-Ended Attention* emerges from the patient's developing *Capacity to Depend*. Where earlier configurations are organized around structure—through rigidity, compliance, or withdrawal—this configuration reflects a shift in the patient's tolerance for openness itself. The impulse to control or resolve begins to loosen, allowing unformulated experience to surface.

This configuration was part of the original surrender model published in *The Process of Opening to Experiencing* (Rickard, 2008), where it appeared under the name *Open* (p. 29). Even then, it marked an inflection point away from defensive closure and toward a mode of engagement grounded in receptivity. In this expanded model, the term *Open-Ended Attention* more precisely captures the psychological orientation required: a sustained willingness to remain with ambiguity, affective nuance, and inner movement without immediate interpretation or resolution.

Its placement is essential. Without a growing tolerance for ambiguity and symbolic uncertainty, the deeper destabilizations characteristic of later capacities—regression, grief, ecstasy—cannot unfold. This configuration does not represent full surrender, but a loosening of the grip. Experience can be held in suspension, allowing meaning to emerge rather than be extracted.

From a metapsychological perspective, this configuration reflects a shift from secondary process dominance toward a more receptive state in which primary process material—unassimilated affect, dream imagery, somatic cues—can be encountered without disorganization. Drawing on Bion's (1967/2014) formulation of no memory, no desire, the therapist's capacity to sustain this openness becomes central to the stability of the analytic field.

*Open-Ended Attention* thus occupies a critical threshold—linking relational trust with an emerging internal spaciousness. While less visibly dramatic than later capacities, it is foundational: the condition under which deeper surrender becomes possible.

## Concluding Reflections

*Open-Ended Attention* marks a shift in how experience itself can be held. What once required structure, explanation, or resolution can now remain in suspension, without immediate closure. This does not eliminate anxiety; rather, it changes the patient's relationship to it.

For both patient and therapist, this configuration requires a sustained tolerance of uncertainty—an ability to remain with what is emerging without prematurely organizing it. In this space, aspects of the self that could not previously be encountered begin to take form, often indirectly, through image, sensation, or fleeting affect.

What develops here is not yet surrender in its fuller sense, but the capacity that makes it possible: a way of attending that does not foreclose experience. From this position, the analytic process can begin to move into deeper and more destabilizing terrain, where what emerges is not only unknown, but transformative.

# 6 The Capacity to Regress

The *Capacity to Regress* marks a turning point in the surrender process. What has been held together through effort, structure, and adaptation begins to loosen, making contact with earlier, more vulnerable states possible. This movement is rarely experienced as relief. For many patients, it brings a sense of instability, as the defenses that once ensured psychological survival can no longer be relied upon in the same way.

What emerges in this regression is not simply memory, but the reappearance of experiences that were never fully lived. As Winnicott (1974) observed, the anxieties encountered in such states are not anticipatory but linked to "a breakdown that has already been experienced" (p. 104). These unformulated agonies remain organized outside of symbolization, held in place by defensive structures that give the appearance of cohesion.

To approach them requires a relinquishing of that cohesion. For some patients, this means loosening a carefully maintained self-reliance; for others, it involves risking a dependence that once felt dangerous or impossible. The fear is not unfounded. Regression can bring with it the sense of losing form—of encountering affect that threatens to overwhelm or disorganize. Yet within a containing analytic relationship, these experiences can begin to take shape, making possible a form of integration that was previously unavailable.

## Gabriella

After a couple of years of steady work, something in Gabriella's way of holding herself began, at times, to give.

She still arrived composed—measured voice, deliberate pacing, the same careful attention to what was said and what was not. But there were moments now when that organization didn't fully hold. A sentence would start and not quite land. A thought would appear without its usual framing, as though her capacity to gather experience into coherent thought had briefly loosened.

"I had a strange feeling this week," she said once, early in the session.

I waited.

DOI: 10.4324/9781003795803-8

"It wasn't exactly… sadness." A pause. "Or maybe it was. I couldn't really tell."

She looked at me briefly, then away, as if unsure what she was asking.

"What was it like, not being able to tell?" I asked.

She hesitated. "Uncomfortable." Another pause. "But also… I don't know… closer to something."

The last phrase seemed to surprise her. She didn't elaborate.

On another day, she arrived and sat down without speaking. This wasn't unusual—but the silence felt different. Less structured. Not withheld, but unformed.

"I almost didn't come," she said eventually.

Then, after a pause: "Not because I didn't want to. More like… I didn't know how to be here today."

I didn't respond immediately.

She shifted slightly in her chair. "That sounds strange."

"It doesn't have to make sense right away," I said.

She nodded but didn't pick the thread back up. The moment passed without being organized into something clearer.

At times, she would begin speaking and stop mid-sentence, as though the thought had dissolved before it could be completed.

"I was thinking about something you said last week and it—" she stopped, frowned slightly, "I don't know where it went."

We sat there together, without trying to recover it.

These were not dramatic changes, but brief suspensions—moments in which Gabriella was less able to organize her experience into coherent thought and affect, and less inclined to restore that organization immediately. What emerged was not regression as collapse, but regression as a temporary loosening of her usual defensive organization: a state in which experience could appear without being quickly structured or contained.

At times, this brought unease.

"I feel a bit… off," she said once. "Like I'm not quite put together the way I usually am."

There was no panic in it, but no reassurance either.

"I think I spend a lot of time making sure I am put together," she added.

We didn't move to interpret. The experience itself was the work.

Regression, for Gabriella, did not mean a return to the past in any explicit form. It appeared in these small shifts—in moments where meaning was not immediately secured, where affect was present but not yet symbolized, and where she could remain in a state of partial unorganization without immediately restoring control.

She did not stay there long. But she no longer avoided it entirely.

## Winston

By the time this phase of the work began to emerge, Winston's life had already become difficult to manage in ways he could no longer dismiss as circumstantial.

He arrived one evening irritated, but not in the usual way. There was a strain to it—less performative, less contained.

"They're still there," he said, dropping into the chair. "I told you about them. The couple."

I nodded.

"They had another fight last night. Loud. Woke me up at two." He shook his head. "I should've kicked them out weeks ago."

He paused, then added, "I almost did."

"What stopped you?" I asked.

He looked at me, then away. "I don't know. It just... didn't happen."

The irritation didn't organize into anything clearer. It lingered, unfocused.

A few minutes later, he said, "I didn't go into work today."

That was new.

"I just... stayed home. Couldn't deal with it." He rubbed his forehead. "The house was a mess. They were still asleep. I just sat there."

"What was that like?" I asked.

He frowned. "I don't know. Stupid." A pause. "I should've done something."

We sat with it.

"I kept thinking I'd get up," he continued. "Clean something. Make coffee. Call someone. But I didn't." Another pause. "I just sat there."

His tone shifted slightly—not quite flat, not quite distressed. Something less organized.

"Felt like I couldn't move," he said, almost as an afterthought. "Not physically. Just... didn't."

I didn't respond.

He glanced at me, as if expecting something, then looked down again.

"That doesn't make any sense," he added.

We stayed there.

Over the following sessions, similar moments appeared. Not as stories he told cleanly, but as fragments—half-formed accounts, interrupted sequences, things that didn't quite link together.

"I had this thought yesterday—" he began once, then stopped. "No, it's gone."

Another time: "I was driving and I almost... I don't know. Missed the turn, I guess. Or didn't care if I did."

He would often circle back, trying to make sense of it, but the organizing thread didn't fully return.

What had once been managed through action—through taking people in, fixing things, staying in motion—was no longer organizing his experience in the same way. But what emerged in its place was not clarity. It was a stalled state in which intention, action, and feeling no longer aligned, and could not be brought back into alignment through effort alone.

At times, this brought flashes of frustration.

"I don't get why I don't just fix it," he said once. "It's not complicated."

But the statement didn't restore anything. It landed without conviction.

In these moments, Winston's usual way of organizing experience—through external action and the creation of dependency around him—had begun to loosen. What emerged was not insight, but a state he could not fully direct, and could not easily escape.

He did not collapse. But he could no longer maintain himself through doing.

We remained with it, without moving too quickly to restore what had begun to loosen.

## Tinsley

Tinsley never approached the door of regression—not because she didn't need care, but because needing care threatened her structure. Her defenses weren't soft—they were tight, spinning, elegant. Obsessive loops disguised as clarity. Armor framed as insight. Her suffering arrived well-articulated, never experienced.

Once, after describing a panic attack she had on a plane, she immediately launched into a theory about attachment trauma and the nervous system. "It's fine, though," she said. "It's just physiology. I know how to regulate it now."

Any hint of dependency was converted into cognition before it could enter the field.

With Tinsley, the atmosphere was sharp-edged, fast-moving. Nothing was allowed to slow down enough to spill.

Regression in her world wasn't repressed—it was evacuated, like something dangerous she had to manage before it contaminated her precision. She didn't resist therapy; she curated it. And in that curation, there was no room for a child self, no trust in the field, no softness that could be allowed to linger.

## What It Asks of the Therapist

Working with regression is not simply about allowing the patient to go backward—it's about the therapist's capacity to stay still when the patient's usual organization begins to loosen. Gabriella, Winston, and Tinsley each approached the threshold of regression differently, and what they revealed was not just the patient's struggle, but the therapist's invitation to surrender to states of uncertainty, ambiguity, and suspended knowing.

With Gabriella, the therapist had to surrender the wish to move things forward. Her vulnerability arrived in subtle glimmers—small disruptions in a long-standing structure of self-containment. To meet her there, the therapist had to let go of the desire to interpret, to illuminate, to offer coherence. Instead, what was required was something more elemental: a steady presence, a reverie-like attention that allowed fragments of affect to emerge without being quickly organized. The therapist had to tolerate the slow pace, the partial nature of the regression, and the pull to stabilize what had only just begun to loosen.

With Winston, regression took on a different weight. It did not appear primarily as symbolization, but as a disruption in his capacity to organize himself through action. The therapist had to surrender the expectation that sessions would feel coherent or productive. At times, the room filled with inertia, fragmentation, and the quiet pressure to restore movement—to suggest, to direct, to make something happen. Here, the task was to remain with a state in which intention, action, and feeling no longer aligned, without stepping in to reconstitute that alignment prematurely. The therapist's own responses—feelings of futility, urgency, or even disengagement—had to be registered without being enacted. Presence, in this context, was not passive, but a refusal to organize the patient's experience on his behalf.

Tinsley, in contrast, demanded a different kind of surrender. She did not regress—not because she couldn't, but because regression would have exposed a need she could not survive. For the therapist, this meant surrendering the expectation that regression is a universal pathway. It required recognizing the defensive necessity of her structure and resisting the pull to break through it. The task was not to induce regression, but to work within the limits of what could be tolerated—accepting that the work might remain organized, cognitive, and externally oriented. That too is a form of holding.

Across these cases, what is asked of the therapist is a disciplined restraint—an ability to remain emotionally receptive without becoming intrusive, to stay engaged without directing, and to tolerate states that do not immediately organize into meaning.

Where regression begins to emerge, this demand intensifies. It challenges the therapist to relinquish the need for progress, clarity, or emotional reciprocity, and to remain present in states where the patient may be opaque, disorganized, or not yet symbolizing experience.

To contain regression is not to guide it or resolve it. It is to sustain a holding environment in which less organized states can be experienced without being immediately structured. The therapist must tolerate this temporality—resisting the pull to move the work forward—and trust that what appears as a loss of organization may be a necessary condition for transformation.

## Justification for the Placement of this Configuration

The *Capacity to Regress* holds a necessary place as the fourth configuration in the surrender model. It represents a crucial turning point, allowing patients to begin accessing, confronting, and metabolizing dissociated emotional states that could not be integrated within earlier configurations. As Donald Winnicott (1974) wrote, the fear of regression is often the fear of a breakdown that has already happened—an early psychic wound that was never emotionally experienced in full.

Gabriella's slow, tentative loosening of control illustrates how regression does not arrive as dramatic collapse, but as moments in which experience is no longer fully organized or held in its usual form. What emerges is not simply dependency, but a state in which affect is present without being immediately structured—where something previously contained can begin to appear without being managed. In Winston, we see a different form: regression arriving through a disruption in his capacity to organize himself through action, as if the structures that once held him in place no longer function in the same way. These expressions of regression—whether subtle or more destabilizing—offer a chance to reintegrate dissociated states within a containing therapeutic relationship.

Even Tinsley, whose obsessive defenses and polished self-presentation keep regression at bay, helps illustrate its significance. Her refusal to allow unprocessed experience into the room underscores just how much is at stake in this configuration. Regression, when possible, becomes not just a descent—but a return to something that once lacked witness.

## Concluding Reflections

The *Capacity to Regress* is foundational in the surrender process—not because it appears cleanly or predictably, but because it allows previously unexperienced emotional states to enter the therapeutic field. It is not a configuration every patient can access. For some, like Tinsley, regression remains out of reach; yet even this refusal reveals how the psyche organizes itself around what cannot yet be felt.

The configurations described thus far establish the psychological conditions that make surrender possible. What follows moves beyond preparation, into the metabolizing of what emerges once that destabilization can be endured.

# Part II

# Releasement Level A

## Deepening Surrender

### *The Body's Integrative Systems*[1]

After the groundwork of the foundational configurations has been laid—the *Closed* state, *Capacity to Depend, Open-Ended Attention*, and *Capacity to Regress*—the surrender process takes on a different character. These next configurations reflect a shift: no longer organized primarily around psychic survival, experience begins to be engaged more symbolically, relationally, and representationally.

This level of the model, *Releasement Level A*—comprising *Capacity to Contain, Readiness for Anxiety, Capacity to Accept Reality, Tolerance of Frustration, Capacity to Symbolize, Subjective Appropriation, Discipline Not to Reason, Suffering Necessary for Transformation, Purification (Catharsis)*, and *Preparation for Love*—functions like the integrative systems of the body: the nervous system, digestive system, and endocrine feedback loops. They are associated with attunement, regulation, and the capacity to metabolize difficult experience.

In this tier, surrender is no longer only about safety—it is about contact, meaning-making, and affect tolerance. These capacities do not appear in isolation. They are associated with therapeutic encounter, with repeated return to earlier themes, and with the presence of psychic space in which complexity can be borne. This configuration is often present in instances where the psyche is able to withstand the reorganizing force of the experiences that follow.

Neurobiologically, this level is associated with coordination between the brain regions involved in affect regulation and reflective function—particularly circuits connecting the limbic system with the prefrontal cortex. In contexts where the nervous system is more regulated within relational experience, there may be greater access to symbolic thinking, emotional modulation, and the capacity to make meaning from affective experience. These integrative processes can be understood as contributing to the physiological conditions associated with psychic depth, making it more possible to hold contradiction, endure frustration, and begin to transform suffering into understanding.

## Note

1 The bodily systems named in the Releasement levels are used metaphorically, not anatomically. They evoke the rhythm, function, and psychic tone associated with each configuration of surrender, rather than implying physiological causation.

DOI: 10.4324/9781003795803-9

# 7 The Capacity to Contain

With the emergence of more primitive emotional states, a new demand takes shape: the need to remain with what arises without being overwhelmed by it. What was previously defended against or avoided now presses more insistently into experience, often with a force that threatens to disorganize the patient's psychic organization.

The *Capacity to Contain* does not eliminate this intensity. Rather, it allows the patient to hold it—to remain in contact with affect that might otherwise provoke escape, fragmentation, or defensive retreat. In this sense, containment becomes a necessary condition for surrender: without it, what is encountered cannot be endured.

To contain is not to control or suppress, but to sustain a psychological space in which experience can unfold without immediate action or collapse. It is this capacity that allows inner turmoil to be approached, rather than evaded, and gradually given form.

## Understanding Containment

Containment, as articulated by Bion (1962), refers to the therapist's capacity to receive and hold the patient's unprocessed emotional experience. What enters the analytic space is often not yet thinkable—affect that arrives without form, coherence, or symbolic representation. Through the therapist's capacity to bear and remain with these states, something begins to shift: what was overwhelming may gradually become tolerable, and what could not be thought may begin to take shape.

This process does not eliminate emotional intensity. Rather, it makes it possible to remain in contact with it without disorganization or defensive retreat. Over time, the patient may begin to internalize this function, developing the capacity to hold experience without needing to evacuate, act upon, or resolve it prematurely.

DOI: 10.4324/9781003795803-10

## Winston

At first glance, Winston's tendency to let strangers live in his home and his disregard for basic hygiene might have seemed like eccentricity—or misdirected compassion. But in therapy, it became clear these were forms of unconscious self-sabotage and disavowed rage. Rather than containing his emotional world, Winston had developed a pattern of externalizing it—allowing the chaos he felt internally to live in his environment and on his body.

In one session, Winston said flatly, "It's like... if everything around me is falling apart, then at least it's not just *me*. I can pretend it's all external."

I stayed quiet, allowing the words to linger.

Then he added, "I don't know how to hold things inside. Guilt, shame, whatever this thing is in my chest—it leaks. It always leaks."

Winston's emotions often felt unmanageable to him—too intense, too shapeless. He lacked the internal containers needed to metabolize difficult affect, and instead, sought to disperse that affect outward. His house became a physical manifestation of his psyche: porous, boundaryless, overrun.

In another session, after describing how one guest had taken advantage of his hospitality, he looked up, his voice hollow. "I don't know why I let them in. I knew he'd steal from me. It's like... I needed him to. To prove something. To make it match."

"Match what?" I asked gently.

He hesitated, then whispered, "What I think I deserve."

These moments were raw but essential. My role was not to reassure or correct, but to hold the emotional weight with him—to provide psychic containment when he couldn't do it himself. I resisted the pull to interpret too quickly or offer solutions. Instead, I reflected back what I sensed:

"You're trying to build a container out of your surroundings. But what if it's something we can build inside you, together? So that the leaking doesn't feel like drowning."

Over time, Winston became less reactive and more curious. He began to recognize how his behaviors were not acts of generosity, but expressions of disorganized guilt and a deep-seated identification with his mother's passivity and his father's disdain. Through our work, he slowly learned to tolerate affect without acting it out—to sit with painful feelings long enough for them to be held, named, and eventually integrated.

One day, he came in and said, "I cleaned the bathroom." He said it casually, but we both knew what it meant. Something that had long been left to accumulate—both in his home and in himself—was beginning to be taken in hand. He was starting, tentatively, to make internal space—to claim the inside world as his own.

## Bill

He arrived like usual—creased shirt, silent nod, the faint smell of oil and detergent. A man built around the idea of not exploding. The room felt metallic that day. Like static waiting for the ground.

We sat.

I thought about machines. How they don't ask questions. How they hum until they don't.

He spoke first. "She says I'm disappearing."

There was a vibration under the words. Not a feeling, exactly. More like something held in the chest for too long. Pressure without release.

I said nothing. Not yet.

"Last night," he said, "I dropped a glass. It shattered. I just stood there."

I felt the shards, though none were on the floor. There was something in the room that wasn't him, wasn't me—something jagged and still.

He looked at me like he was trying to decide whether I was flammable.

"I get these thoughts. Like, what if I just walked out? Got in the truck. Didn't say anything."

I thought of engines that overheat and stall. Of doors that don't slam, just click shut forever.

"You don't say much," he added. No accusation. Just a reading on the monitor.

"You're bringing something in here that's hard to hold," I said, quietly. "I'm trying not to drop it."

That landed. Or maybe it didn't. But the current shifted.

Silence came next—not empty but charged. Like the silence after a misfire.

Then, softer: "I used to be useful."

Not quite grief. Not quite rage. Something more elemental. A lost function.

We didn't interpret that day. We didn't trace it to his father, or the base, or the years between. We stayed with the hum of something breaking down in slow motion.

That session taught me something about containment I hadn't known: that sometimes, it means keeping the room from overheating. Not with coolness, but with presence. Not muting the fire, but letting it burn where it won't destroy.

Later, he said, "You didn't move that day."

I didn't know which day. But I nodded.

"Good," he said. "I needed that."

## What It Asks of the Therapist

To help a patient develop internal containment, the therapist must first become the container. This is more than a technical stance—it's a psychological and emotional labor that requires the therapist to surrender their own comfort, expectations, and even—at times—their felt sense of vitality.

With Winston, containment meant enduring a slow, ambient unraveling. His shame didn't explode—it leaked. The therapist was required to remain close without smothering, attuned without organizing, still without abandoning. Winston externalized his inner chaos through passivity, neglect, and unconscious self-punishment. To sit with him was to enter a murky atmosphere where nothing catastrophic happened but everything felt on the verge of disintegration.

In contrast, a patient like Bill challenges the therapist in a different way. Where Winston discharges affect quietly, Bill does so through force. He might lash out, raise his voice, or accuse the therapist of not "getting it." His volatility may mask a buried grief, or a collapsed masculinity he refuses to name. In one session, he might accuse the therapist of sounding patronizing. In another, he might abruptly storm out or arrive smelling like alcohol, only to claim he's "fine." His psyche doesn't leak—it *erupts*—and the therapist is asked not to retaliate, not to recoil, but to receive the affect without being shattered by it.

In both cases, the therapist must manage what is being projected into them. Whether it's Winston's deadness or Bill's disorganized rage, these are not simply emotions to be named; they are states of being the therapist is temporarily asked to house. This task is particularly difficult when it triggers countertransference responses—feelings of futility, deadness, boredom, or irritation that echo the patient's inner world.

Winnicott's (1969) three principles for the psychotherapist are especially relevant here:

1 *Be consistent.*
2 *Survive the patient's attacks.*
3 *Stay alive.*

The last of these—*to stay alive*—can be the hardest when working with patients like Winston and Bill. In some sessions, staying alive means resisting the lure of detachment or over-functioning. In others, it means noticing the creeping desire to retaliate, to fall silent, to become emotionally absent. These are signs the therapist is being pulled into what André Green (1983/1993) called the psychic landscape of the *dead mother*—a maternal figure who has emotionally withdrawn, leaving behind a void that the patient either tries to fill with chaos or mirrors with collapse.

The therapist must be able to sense when they are at risk of becoming a *dead object* in the room—a passive recipient of unbearable projections—and choose, again and again, not to disappear. This is the paradox of containment: the therapist must hold what the patient cannot bear, without becoming overwhelmed or emptied in the process. It is a quiet endurance, and it is often the most vital thing the therapist brings.

To surrender to this task is to accept that containment will not always look like understanding or soothing. Sometimes it looks like simply being there—alive, steady, and emotionally available—when the patient fully expects you not to be. Over time, this presence becomes something the patient can internalize. Not all at once. But incrementally, through every moment the therapist chooses to stay alive in the face of what feels unbearable.

## Justification for the Placement of this Configuration

*Capacity to Contain* is placed at this juncture in the surrender model as a pivotal transition from foundational configurations—safety, dependency, open-ended attention—into the more metabolically demanding configurations of psychic transformation. As defenses loosen and receptivity increases, what emerges—grief, rage, shame, desire—requires containment. Without it, the process risks dysregulation rather than transformation.

Containment serves as the bridge between letting go and being able to remain intact during the letting go. It is not simply about tolerating affect; it is about housing it in a way that does not rupture the self. This capacity is essential before a patient can enter into the more destabilizing dimensions of surrender that follow—such as dissolution of self-states, confrontation with unformulated experience, or the deconstruction of prior identifications.

The *Capacity to Contain* is also a cornerstone of the surrender process, as it enables patients to engage with their emotions more fully and authentically. By containing their feelings, patients can experience a deeper sense of self-understanding and resilience. They no longer need to avoid or act out their emotions; instead, they can integrate these experiences, building a more cohesive and stable self. As patients internalize the *Capacity to Contain*, they become better equipped to face the demands of subsequent capacities, where deeper layers of surrender require greater emotional resilience. Containment provides a foundation for these capacities, allowing patients to approach them with a sense of groundedness and self-assurance.

This configuration also signals a shift in the therapeutic field. The therapist no longer simply offers reliability or attunement; they must now become a vessel for unmanageable affect, accepting projections of deadness, volatility, or abandonment without becoming undone themselves. In this way, the work of containment involves not only the patient's growth, but the therapist's own willingness to be used, survived, and ultimately internalized as a containing presence.

Without this configuration, the surrender model would move too quickly into psychic exposure without adequate scaffolding. The chapters that follow will explore more destabilizing or revelatory dimensions of surrender. The *Capacity to Contain* ensures that the patient has developed a psychic interior sturdy enough to encounter those dimensions without collapse.

## Concluding Reflections

The *Capacity to Contain* introduces a new condition in the surrender process: what emerges no longer needs to be expelled, avoided, or acted out, but can be held. Containment does not resolve what emerges—it makes it bearable.

In the chapters that follow, the work deepens. What is held can be encountered more fully, and the patient is asked not only to bear experience, but to remain in contact with it as it unfolds.

# 8 Readiness for Anxiety

There comes a point in the surrender process where what emerges can no longer be met with curiosity alone. It begins to carry a different weight—less interpretable, more unsettling. The patient is no longer simply opening to experience but encountering something that resists being known.

*Readiness for Anxiety* is the capacity to remain in contact with this shift. It is not a passive endurance of discomfort, but a willingness to stay with what disorients—without rushing to organize it, explain it, or make it coherent. Both patient and therapist are drawn toward the unknown, and both must resist the pull to restore certainty too quickly.

In this sense, anxiety is not merely a symptom to be reduced, but a signal that something more fundamental is being approached. Heidegger (1927/1962) understood anxiety as opening onto the "darkness of Being"—a state in which familiar structures fall away. In psychoanalytic terms, this corresponds to the patient's increasing contact with unformulated experience. What matters is not eliminating this anxiety but developing the capacity to remain with it.

This requires a tolerance for ambiguity in both members of the analytic pair. The stance Bion described—an openness unanchored by memory or expectation—takes on a different quality here. It is no longer simply a posture of receptivity, but a way of remaining in contact with experience as it becomes more difficult to bear.

## Winston

Winston rarely spoke about his work as a physician. When he did, it was in passing—brief mentions of patients, clinical routines, or insurance paperwork. But beneath this surface lay a deeper discomfort: a persistent sense that he had never measured up. Not to his colleagues, not to the image of what a 'real doctor' should be—and certainly not to his father, a renowned surgeon who had built a career on precision and discipline.

"I just sort of... drifted into general practice," Winston once said, eyes fixed on the floor. "It wasn't like I had a calling. It was more like... inertia. Like I couldn't imagine doing anything else but also couldn't imagine doing it well."

DOI: 10.4324/9781003795803-11

This quiet confession revealed the deeper anxiety Winston carried—not just about being inadequate, but about being *invisible*. While his father was celebrated and exacting, Winston felt forgettable. He didn't crave praise, but he feared exposure—the possibility that someone might confirm what he already suspected: that he wasn't enough.

Anxiety, for Winston, showed up not as panic but as withdrawal. He numbed himself with routine, avoided supervision, and found ways to work just under the radar. "No one bothers me," he once said. "Which is great, right?" But his laugh was thin. He was haunted by a chronic, low-grade dread—the fear that he'd missed something, done harm, or simply been unnoticed.

In one session, he brought up a patient he'd seen in urgent care the week before—a young woman with chest pain. "It turned out fine," he said. "Musculoskeletal, probably. But I woke up at 3 a.m. thinking I'd missed something. I didn't even examine her as thoroughly as I could have. I just... wanted to get through the shift."

"What was that like, waking up in the middle of the night?" I asked.

He hesitated. "Like someone dropped a stone in my chest."

I waited.

"I kept thinking about my dad. He'd never let something like that slide. He'd check everything. Twice."

"What did you do with that feeling?"

He looked out the window. "Made toast. Went back to sleep. Tried not to think."

This moment clarified the depth of Winston's difficulty with anxiety. He didn't repress it so much as quietly shut the door on it—convincing himself there was nothing inside worth looking at. He had learned to survive by keeping emotional tremors small and contained. But therapy began to open space for something else: the possibility that anxiety was not just a threat, but a signal.

Over time, Winston began to speak of these moments more freely—not always with clarity, but with presence. He didn't try to solve them or shut them down. He learned to notice when his heart was racing or when his chest tightened—and to stay with the feeling just a little longer. Not to fix it. Just to name it.

"That feeling," he said one day, "the 3 a.m. thing... it still shows up. But I don't run from it right away. I just kind of... let it sit in the room with me."

For Winston, this was readiness. Not mastery, but presence—the capacity to feel anxious and not disown it, to experience doubt without collapsing into shame or evasion. It was a quiet triumph, forged not in catharsis, but in the simple act of staying put.

## Jerome

Jerome entered therapy already formulating. A litigator by trade, he was used to identifying problems quickly and building cases around them. Each session was prepared, annotated. Dreams were analyzed in advance, and emotions were often pre-empted by formulations: "I think this is about control," he'd say, as if handing over the conclusion of an argument before I had time to listen.

Anxiety, for Jerome, was something to outsmart.

When it crept in, he moved faster. He intellectualized, problem-solved, reframed. The idea of simply sitting with discomfort seemed wasteful, inefficient—even irresponsible. "I know it's irrational," he once said, speaking of his fear that a client would fire him. "So why let it take up space? What good does it do?"

In one session, he described a dream where he was driving through heavy fog. "I couldn't see anything," he said. "And I kept checking the GPS, but it just said: recalculating. Over and over. No directions. Just that."

He smiled faintly. "So, clearly, this is about uncertainty and my current caseload. My mind can't plan. That's the message."

I nodded, then asked, "And what was it like in the dream—the feeling of driving with no visibility?"

He hesitated. "I don't know. Frustrating? Maybe scary. But mostly—I just wanted it to stop."

I didn't interpret. We let the fog hang for a moment.

This was the work—helping Jerome experience anxiety without metabolizing it into language too quickly. He had spent most of his life managing discomfort through brilliance. But brilliance can also be a defense.

Later, he said, "It's like there's a gap between when I feel something and when I explain it. And I always rush to fill the gap."

"What if you didn't?" I asked.

He looked at me—wary, but curious.

Readiness, for Jerome, wasn't about tolerating panic. It was about tolerating not knowing. Not resolving. Letting the fog stay in the dream a little longer. Letting his emotional GPS stutter without rushing for a better route.

He began to notice his impulse to frame everything, and instead, occasionally paused. Breathed. Asked, "What's here if I don't name it yet?"

Over time, those gaps got wider. Not in a dissociative way—but in a spacious one. Room for feeling. Room for presence. Not conclusion, but contact.

## What It Asks of the Therapist

Winston and Jerome present two opposing challenges to a therapist's own readiness for anxiety. Winston retreats from feeling, barely letting it surface. Jerome moves too quickly to control it, packaging discomfort into neat formulations. To support both, the therapist must embody a third stance: one that neither avoids nor resolves anxiety but makes room for it.

This requires the therapist to surrender the need to be helpful in obvious ways. With Winston, that might mean tolerating long silences or low-energy sessions without rushing to enliven the space. With Jerome, it might mean resisting the urge to interpret or affirm too quickly—allowing ambiguity to linger, even when the patient wants answers.

In both cases, the therapist's ability to sit with *unresolved tension* becomes a model. It shows that anxiety need not be evacuated or solved—it can be endured, explored, and even transformed.

This stance demands the therapist manage their own countertransference: the pull to 'fix', to explain, or to withdraw. Anxiety in the room often stirs anxiety in the therapist. But by staying emotionally present and grounded, the therapist shows the patient another way: a path through discomfort that begins not with solutions, but with staying.

## Justification for Placement within Releasement Level A

*Readiness for Anxiety* serves as a preparatory configuration within *Releasement Level A*, making it essential to this level of the surrender model. It builds on the patient's developing capacity for containment and opens into subsequent capacities such as the *Capacity to Accept Reality*. Here, anxiety is no longer treated as an obstacle, but as a necessary condition of self-discovery.

The inclusion of this configuration makes possible the patient's encounter with psychic material that would otherwise remain out of reach. *Readiness for Anxiety* allows what is emerging to be endured rather than avoided. Drawn from the original dissertation research and informed by Heidegger (1927/1962) and Bion (1962), this configuration situates anxiety as a necessary condition of psychological growth.

## Concluding Reflections

Something changes here. What was previously held can no longer remain neutral. It begins to press, to unsettle, to resist being shaped into understanding. The patient is no longer simply containing experience but encountering what strains that capacity.

*Readiness for Anxiety* is what allows this shift to be endured. Not by mastering it, and not by resolving it, but by remaining in contact with what cannot yet be known. What follows will ask more of this capacity—not just to bear experience, but to stay with it as it begins to take on a form that cannot be controlled.

# 9 The Capacity to Accept Reality

There comes a point in the surrender process where what has been sensed, endured, or circled around can no longer remain unacknowledged. What was once held at a distance begins to take on a more definite shape—less ambiguous, more binding. The patient is no longer only approaching experience but encountering something that cannot be deferred.

The *Capacity to Accept Reality* emerges here. It is not simply the recognition of what is true, but the ability to remain in contact with it without retreating into distortion, denial, or omission. What is encountered may not be new; what changes is the patient's capacity to bear it.

At this point, loss begins to register, though not in a uniform or immediately recognizable way. For some patients, there is an emerging awareness that something is being grieved, even where it cannot yet be named or known. This recognition reflects a degree of psychic contact that allows loss to be approached without being fully taken up. Elsewhere, grief does not appear in this form at all. Experience may be felt, enacted, or displaced without becoming available as loss, not because it is being withheld, but because it has not yet taken shape in a way that can be borne. In other instances, the organization of the self continues to operate against such contact, maintaining forms of control, activity, or relational distance that prevent the recognition of loss and limit. What is at stake in these movements is not only the avoidance of pain, but the relinquishment of fantasy—particularly those forms of omnipotence that sustain the possibility that what has been lost might be restored or undone. To accept reality is therefore to come into relation with what cannot be reversed, and with it, the conditions under which grief may begin to register. Where this does not occur, it is not the absence of grief that is observed, but the absence of a form through which it could be lived.

This shift often involves the collapse of illusions that once protected the self. Omnipotent fantasies—of control, exception, or undoing—lose their hold, making room for grief, limitation, and dependency. What follows is not resolution, but a different relation to truth: one that can be lived with rather than avoided.

From a Fairbairnian perspective, the difficulty lies not in recognizing reality, but in relinquishing the internal object relations that protect the

DOI: 10.4324/9781003795803-12

individual from it. Even painful or depriving internal objects may be preferred over the uncertainty of the external world. To accept reality, then, is not simply to see more clearly, but to let go of what has made psychic survival possible—an act that often carries the weight of loss.

What must be surrendered is not only illusion, but the sense of safety it once provided. This difficulty—of relinquishing what protects the psyche from reality—has been approached from multiple vantage points within psychoanalytic theory.

## Understanding the Capacity to Accept Reality

The acceptance of reality occupies a central place in psychoanalytic theory, though it has been approached from different vantage points. Freud (1911) framed it as the movement from wish-fulfillment toward the reality principle, requiring the relinquishment of omnipotent fantasy. Winnicott (1965) located this shift in the process of disillusionment, where the individual comes to face limitation, dependency, and loss as conditions of being.

Bion extended this further, emphasizing not simply the recognition of reality, but the capacity to remain in contact with what has not yet taken form. His adaptation of Keats's notion of negative capability—remaining in "uncertainties, mysteries, doubts" without premature resolution—points to a mode of engagement that precedes understanding. In this state, reality is not grasped but stayed with.

What is encountered at this point is difficult to name directly. In Dante's *Inferno* (Canto III), the line inscribed above the gate— "Abandon all hope, ye who enter here"—is often taken as a sentence of despair, but psychologically it names something far more familiar. The figures in the Inferno are not tortured by external forces; they remain bound to the very illusions that once protected them. Their suffering is organized around omnipotent fantasies they cannot relinquish. In this sense, the inscription is not a command to give up authentic hope, but a warning that hope built on denial or magical undoing cannot accompany one into reality. What must be surrendered is not the possibility of transformation, but the defensive hope that fantasy can spare us from truth. Dante captures the moment when illusion collapses and the psyche stands at the edge of what must be faced—precisely the threshold required in this configuration of surrender.

The acceptance of reality, then, is not passive resignation. It is an active and often painful psychic labor—one that asks the individual to relinquish illusion, encounter grief, and live with what can no longer be undone.

## Gabriella

Gabriella sat with her arms crossed, eyes fixed on a corner of the room.

"I don't need anyone," she said flatly. "I've always been fine on my own."

I let the silence linger. "Fine... or safe?" I asked.

Gabriella's jaw tightened. "Safe, I guess. People always want something, and needing them—" she shrugged, "it's never been worth it."

This was familiar. Gabriella often spoke in polished phrases, presenting herself as self-contained, but beneath it was something more brittle. Having grown up in a controlling household, she had relied on forms of omnipotent fantasy to maintain a sense of coherence when reality felt too exposing.

"Sometimes," I said, "it sounds like being entirely self-reliant was what kept things from falling apart."

Gabriella's posture shifted slightly. She glanced at me, her expression more guarded than before. "Yeah," she said. "I used to make things up... like if I imagined it differently, it wouldn't hurt as much."

I nodded. "And did it?"

She exhaled, the breath catching. "It helped." A pause. "At the time."

We sat with that.

"But now..." she added, more quietly, "I think I just ended up... by myself."

The words didn't fully land, as if she wasn't sure what she was saying yet. I didn't move to clarify.

After a moment, she said, almost to herself, "It's not the same, imagining it."

I met her gaze but didn't add anything.

Gabriella didn't look away. For someone organized around self-sufficiency, remaining in contact without restoring the illusion marked a shift—not toward dependence, but toward a growing tolerance for what is.

## Tinsley

Accepting reality in therapy is rarely mutual. Often, it is the patient who determines what can be acknowledged, while the therapist bears the weight of what remains unspoken. The task is not only to invite recognition, but to withstand the patient's refusal.

Tinsley entered therapy with an air of control and certainty, yet beneath this lay a persistent avoidance of responsibility. There was a pattern in how she related to limits—external structures were tolerated only insofar as they could be managed or reinterpreted. When the continuity of our work was disrupted, I raised it—not as a correction, but as an invitation to consider what it meant for the therapy to be interrupted.

Days later, she ended the treatment. There was no discussion, no attempt at understanding—only a brief message and then absence.

In reflecting on the rupture, it became possible to consider that leaving may have functioned as a way to pre-empt an experience she could not bear. The timing suggested a pattern in which separation was enacted rather than thought, with agency difficult to hold as her own and instead experienced as originating in the other.

Therapy had often unfolded as a one-sided negotiation, where meaning and consequence were difficult for her to sustain internally. When aspects of reality came into view—even without judgment—they were experienced as intrusion. What was offered in the room did not remain as it was given but became reorganized within her internal world.

For some patients, departure does not end the transference—it shifts its location. What cannot be thought may return later, fixed in grievance or certainty, detached from the relational context in which it first emerged.

There was no opportunity for repair. The work ended where it could not be thought.

But rupture, too, belongs to the process. Some structures foreclose reflection altogether. In these cases, the task is not to resolve what cannot be resolved but to bear what the patient cannot hold—to metabolize what was left behind, and to recognize that even this has meaning.

## What It Asks of the Therapist

To help patients develop the capacity to accept reality, the therapist must tolerate what the patient cannot yet bear to know. This is not a matter of presenting truth, but of holding space for it—without intrusion, without withdrawal. The therapist remains at the edge of what the patient avoids, steady, receptive, and non-coercive.

This requires what Bion (1962/1970) described as maternal reverie: the capacity to receive and metabolize unconscious projections without reacting to them. The therapist encounters not only the patient's narrative, but their refusal—what is silenced, deflected, or displaced. Here, the work is often asymmetrical: the therapist must carry what is disavowed without retaliating, interpreting prematurely, or insisting on contact.

Gabriella's case illustrates what becomes possible when this stance is sustained. Her retreat into omnipotent fantasy—shaped by the unreliability of her early relational world—initially resisted interpretation. She dismissed dependency, disavowed longing, and avoided memory. I did not challenge the fantasy directly. Instead, I waited, bore the silences, and remained emotionally available without insistence. Over time, something began to shift. She was able to approach the possibility that the fantasy had protected her—but not without cost. What emerged was not a fully formed recognition, but a growing contact with the fact that what had once held her together had also kept her apart. She began to give voice to what had long remained unsaid, though not always clearly or consistently. My task was not to dismantle the defense, but to remain present without being threatened by it or drawn into it.

Tinsley's departure reflects a different limit. It was not a failure of the therapy, nor of Tinsley herself, but the expression of a structure that could not tolerate certain forms of recognition. The capacity to take up her own experience as her own remained out of reach—not by refusal, but by necessity. When rupture appeared, she did what she had always needed to do: leave before meaning could take shape. For her, the safest reality was one that could be located outside herself. My task was to remain steady in the face of this movement, without forcing contact or attempting to retrieve what she could not hold, even as the work moved beyond reach.

Encounters such as these invite reflection not only on the analytic process, but on the structures patients bring with them. A patient does not enter therapy with a single problem, but with a whole organization of mind—one that may defend against recognition, rupture, and change. It is this structure, as much as any symptom, that shapes what becomes possible in the work. Some treatments place considerable demands on the therapist's internal resources, but strength alone is not sufficient. Where there is a mismatch between the patient's organization and what the therapist can contain—whether temperamentally or theoretically—the work may devolve into impasse or enactment. This is not a matter of blame, but of psychic compatibility and realistic therapeutic limits.

When therapy ends in rejection, the asymmetry of the therapeutic relationship becomes stark. The therapist cannot respond, clarify, or offer context, even when misrepresented. What may present itself as fact can also be understood as a psychological document—an expression of what could not be metabolized within the treatment. For some patients, casting the therapist as persecutor stabilizes the self when agency cannot be borne. For the therapist, this requires not only restraint, but a tolerance for misrecognition—an ethical position that is both silent and exposed.

Across these cases, the therapist's task remains constant: to offer a mind that stays steady amid flight, rupture, or fantasy. One patient, over time, came to recognize that presence and use it as a foothold toward change. The other could not—not through refusal, but through structural necessity. Still, the work holds: to keep open a space where reality may be entered—or, when it cannot, to bear what remains outside it.

## The Role of Helplessness and Dependence in Reality Acceptance

Accepting reality inevitably brings the patient into contact with helplessness and dependence—states that are often experienced as threatening, particularly for those organized around self-reliance or omnipotent control. As these defenses loosen, moments of regression may emerge, allowing a previously warded-off vulnerability to surface.

The therapist's task is not only to tolerate the patient's dependence, but also to bear their own helplessness when the work stalls or when emotional needs cannot be met. This requires remaining present without retreating into interpretation or pressing toward resolution.

In sustaining this position, the therapist offers something more than understanding: a lived experience of dependence that does not shame, and of helplessness that does not collapse. Over time, this makes possible a different relation to limitation—one in which what cannot be controlled need not be disavowed.

## Justification for the Placement of This Configuration

The *Capacity to Accept Reality* marks a decisive point within *Releasement Level A*. Before a patient can work with unconscious material or withstand the disorganizing effects of psychic frustration, they must come into contact with their own experience as it is—not as it has been managed, distorted, or disavowed. This is not a matter of cognitive recognition, but of an affective encounter with what has been avoided.

For this reason, this configuration is not only structurally necessary, but foundational. Without the ability to remain in contact with reality, later capacities—tolerating frustration, sustaining thought under pressure, or engaging symbolic life—cannot take hold in a meaningful way. The work risks becoming either defensive or abstract, rather than transformative.

Reality acceptance functions as a hinge. It does not eliminate defense, but loosens it, creating space for a different relation to experience—one in which the patient can begin to stay with what is, rather than retreat from it. From here, the work can deepen: what has been encountered can be thought, felt, and eventually integrated.

## Concluding Reflections

The *Capacity to Accept Reality* is not a momentary achievement but an evolving psychic position—one that must be revisited as new material emerges. In some patients, it opens the possibility of relational presence, allowing long-buried truths to enter the room without collapse. In others, contact with reality remains too destabilizing, prompting flight or projection. In both, the therapist's task is not to enforce reality, but to inhabit it—to remain anchored when the patient cannot.

This configuration establishes a relation to truth that is neither annihilating nor idealized. Without it, symbolic elaboration risks becoming dissociative and tolerance of frustration remains abstract. Here, the work takes hold: what has been feared or denied can be named, held, and eventually lived.

# 10 Tolerance of Frustration

*Tolerance of Frustration* is a pivotal configuration within *Releasement Level A*, defined by the patient's capacity to endure unmet desire, unresolved affect, and the uncertainty inherent in the work. Without it, emotional pain and limitation are managed through defense or avoidance. *Tolerance of Frustration* makes possible the development of deeper thinking, symbolic processing, and, ultimately, psychic growth.

## Understanding Tolerance of Frustration

In psychoanalytic theory, frustration refers to the experience of an unmet desire, often accompanied by a range of painful emotions such as anxiety, despair, and hopelessness. Bion emphasized that frustration is a necessary ingredient for mental growth. For Bion, frustration creates a gap between the desire and its fulfillment, and it is within this gap that the capacity to think develops. When frustration is tolerated, the mind can begin to process raw emotions and transform them into meaningful thoughts, allowing for the development of insight and resilience.

This tolerance for frustration is rooted in early experiences. Bion (1962) highlighted the significance of an infant's encounter with frustration, such as when a caregiver is not immediately available to satisfy a need. If the infant can tolerate the absence of gratification, they can start to form an understanding of their inner world and reality. However, if the frustration is intolerable, the infant may turn to defensive mechanisms, such as omnipotent fantasy, hallucinations, or aggressive reactions, which distort their perception of reality and impede psychic growth.

## Gabriella

Gabriella entered each session with a controlled formality—posture straight, voice composed, blouse neatly tucked. A retired schoolteacher, she spoke with the diction of someone who had long relied on composure as protection. Her words often arrived polished, but just behind them something less contained pressed forward: a pause that lingered, a breath held slightly too

DOI: 10.4324/9781003795803-13

long. Her frustration was rarely expressed directly. It appeared in small shifts—the tightening of her jaw, a glance away mid-sentence—as if she sensed something emerging that she could not fully allow.

She did not name envy easily. When it appeared, it came out indirectly, and often with a trace of dismissal.

"It must be nice," she said. "To not be the one who cares more."

Her expression did not change.

I did not move to reassure or clarify. "It sounds like something in that feels difficult to hold on your own," I said.

She paused, then shook her head slightly. "It's not that. It's just the way people are."

I let the silence remain.

After a moment, I said, "Maybe there's a part of you that expects disappointment… and another part that still feels it."

She shifted in her seat. "I don't think about it like that."

There was a tightening in her voice now—subtle, but present.

I didn't press further. The feeling was there, but not yet something she could take up directly.

"You always do that," she said after a moment. "Try to make it into something."

I let that stand.

"I think something is there," I said. "But we don't have to settle it right now."

She looked at me briefly, then away again.

"You're not the first person I've envied," she said, more quietly. "But you're the first one I didn't leave because of it."

The words seemed to arrive before she had decided to say them.

I stayed with what she had offered, without expanding it.

"It matters that you stayed," I said.

She gave a small nod, almost imperceptible.

"That's different," she said.

The envy did not resolve, nor did the frustration become easier. But it no longer required immediate dismissal or retreat. She could remain in contact with it for longer stretches, even as it unsettled her. And I became someone she did not have to idealize—or move away from—to continue.

## Winston

Winston's sessions felt heavy before he even spoke. The air seemed denser when he entered the room, as though he carried something that lingered behind him. A GP, he spoke in a low voice, sometimes barely audible, as though he were unsure he should be heard. There was often the sense that he had just missed something—arriving a moment too late or standing somewhere he wasn't sure he belonged. He came in with coffee stains on his coat, sometimes smelling faintly of mildew or cologne—never the same scent twice.

In session, his frustration rarely appeared as complaint. It showed up in evasions, in a slow detour around anything emotionally precise. If something came too close, he would pivot.

"Did I tell you about the neighbor's dog? Keeps dragging trash into my yard," he said once after I named a pattern of self-neglect.

I didn't follow the detour. "You shift away when something gets close," I said. "I'm wondering what made that harder to stay with just now."

He stared at the floor. "You sound like my old supervisor. She used to say that." A pause. "I hated that."

I waited.

"It's okay if you hate it in me too," I said.

That landed. He didn't respond right away, but he didn't shift the subject either. The silence took on shape, something neither of us moved to interrupt.

Eventually, he said, "You know what's worse? I actually miss her now."

I didn't draw it out. With Winston, meaning had to gather slowly; anything more forceful risked losing him.

Another time, after several missed appointments, he returned looking disheveled and out of breath.

"Sorry," he said, though it was unclear what for. "My head's been... not where it should be."

I didn't ask where his head had been. "You came back," I said.

He looked at me, half-suspicious. "Wasn't sure I would."

"That makes sense," I said. "Sometimes it's easier not to come back."

He let out a faint, almost inaudible laugh. "Yeah."

There was no dramatic turn. But over time, he didn't leave the moment as quickly when something pressed in. He still wandered, still deflected, but at times he would pause, as if registering it while it was happening.

"I'm doing it again," he said once, trailing off. "Talking around it."

"Yes," I said. "And you're still here."

What changed wasn't the frustration—it was his ability to remain in contact with it, even briefly, without moving away. I held his evasions, his irritability, his shame without forcing them into meaning too quickly. That steadiness made more presence possible. It wasn't that Winston stopped zig-zagging. It was that, at times, he no longer disappeared inside it.

## What It Asks of the Therapist

As Bion (1962) observed, frustration is not just something to be endured—it is the psychic space where thought begins. Here, the therapist must function as an alpha function: taking in raw, unformulated experience and returning it in a form that can be borne and eventually thought.

Working with frustration is not about teaching patience—it is about holding the structure of a patient who cannot yet tolerate absence, lack, or longing without collapse or retaliation. The therapist becomes a kind of scaffold, able to absorb projections of deprivation, envy, and disappointment without resolving them too quickly or retreating from them. What the patient cannot yet bear must be held, thought about, and returned in a form that can be used.

With Winston, this meant remaining inside a kind of disorganization, where frustration did not appear as complaint but as drift and misdirection. My task was not to interrupt this, but to stay close to it without becoming absorbed by it. I had to offer a kind of psychic friction—enough to be felt, not so much as to be avoided. Not following the detours, returning to what had just been left: "You shift away when something gets close." And, at times, simply marking continuity: "You came back." This stance allowed Winston, at moments, to register frustration rather than move past it, and to remain in contact with it without disappearing.

Gabriella required something different: an encounter with envy that was controlled, precise, and difficult for her to take up directly. Her frustration emerged in the experience of caring more, of feeling without response, and in the pressure to disavow that imbalance. She approached this indirectly—"It must be nice... to not be the one who cares more"—and could just as quickly move away from it. To work with her, I had to remain steady in the face of that asymmetry, without softening it or making it easier to bear. Envy could not be exposed too directly or interpreted too soon. Instead, it had to be allowed to appear in fragments, and to be taken up only as far as she could hold it: "You're not the first person I've envied... but you're the first I didn't leave because of it." My task was to remain present without demand, and to tolerate the tension between contact and withdrawal.

Both patients make clear that frustration tolerance is not built through insight alone, but through sustained, regulated contact. The therapist must know when to speak and when to wait—when to name something precisely, and when to leave it partially unformed. Whether it appears as drift or critique, evasion or restraint, frustration asks the therapist to remain present without retaliating or withdrawing. It is this survival that gradually allows the patient to discover that frustration need not rupture the relationship.

## Justification for the Placement of This Configuration

*Tolerance of Frustration* precedes the *Capacity to Symbolize* in *Releasement Level A* because it functions like connective tissue within the psyche's representational system. Just as ligaments must absorb tension to allow for movement without rupture, the mind must be able to withstand emotional strain in order to support the formation of symbolic thought. When frustration cannot be tolerated, the psyche responds as if under threat—mobilizing defenses that constrict experience and restrict access to meaning. But when frustration is endured, even in small doses, it creates a kind of psychic elasticity. This elasticity allows emotionally charged experience to be metabolized rather than expelled, making space for symbols to emerge and for inner life to be expressed with coherence and depth.

This sequence reflects Bion's (1962) belief that the capacity to think develops in response to frustration. By enduring the gap between desire and satisfaction, patients begin to think and reflect on their experience, transforming raw emotion into something that can be known.

When frustration cannot be tolerated, this process collapses. The object cannot be held in mind as both needed and disappointing. Instead of thinking, the patient evacuates; instead of remaining, contact is disrupted—internally or relationally. The therapist may be idealized or attacked, experienced as withholding, punitive, or cold. What might have generated thought instead generates distortion.

In relational terms, intolerance of frustration destabilizes the possibility of surrender. If the patient cannot remain in contact with an object who disappoints or fails to gratify, the work of integration halts. Ambivalence becomes intolerable, and the object must either be preserved as perfect or rejected altogether.

Frustration tolerance determines whether the patient can remain in relationship when unmet need emerges. In Gabriella's earlier patterns, moments of envy were difficult to sustain and often led to withdrawal before they could be taken up. In Winston, frustration gave way to misdirection and inertia, with emotional contact slipping out of reach when it became too immediate. In both cases, the inability to tolerate frustration placed strain on the continuity of the relationship. The therapeutic task was not to eliminate frustration, but to make it survivable.

Without this capacity, surrender cannot deepen. The patient cannot remain long enough in the gap between desire and reality for symbolization to occur. Thought collapses under pressure, contact ruptures, and what might have become meaning is instead expelled.

## Concluding Reflections

*Tolerance of Frustration* marks a consolidation within *Releasement Level A*. It allows patients to remain in contact with unmet desire and unresolved emotional tension without collapsing into distortion or withdrawal. It is the first sustained experience of staying with an object who does not immediately gratify, repair, or clarify. For patients like Winston and Gabriella, this meant beginning to discover that disappointment need not destroy the relationship. Frustration could be felt—and, at times, survived.

This capacity becomes a turning point in the surrender process. It makes possible the emergence of symbolic thinking. Without the ability to remain in the gap between desire and reality, symbolization cannot take hold. When frustration can be borne, emotionally charged experience becomes available for representation rather than evacuation. Thought begins to take the place of distortion.

In the chapters that follow, this capacity supports the development of symbolization, subjective appropriation, and deeper psychic transformation. With frustration tolerance established, the patient can remain in relationship—and in thought—long enough for something new to form.

# 11 The Capacity to Symbolize

The *Capacity to Symbolize* emerges as a central development within *Releasement Level A*. It allows raw emotional experience to take form—no longer overwhelming or undifferentiated, but able to be represented, reflected upon, and gradually understood. Through symbolization, what was previously unthinkable becomes available to thought. This capacity creates the conditions for deeper surrender, as patients begin to engage their inner world rather than evacuate or enact it.

## Understanding the Capacity to Symbolize

Symbolization introduces distance. It allows an experience to stand for something, rather than be confused with it. Without this capacity, emotional life remains concrete—felt but not thought about. When symbolization becomes possible, patients can begin to hold their experience in mind, rather than act it out or become overwhelmed by it.

This distinction is captured clearly in Hanna Segal's (1957) work on symbol formation, the distinction between symbol and symbolic equation is central. She writes of a patient who played a string instrument and experienced a disturbing confusion between the sensual, expressive act of playing and literal masturbation. Rather than recognizing the instrument as symbolically linked to unconscious sexual fantasy, he experienced the act as equivalent to it. The instrument did not represent—it was.

This is what Segal termed a symbolic equation: the collapse of distance between symbol and thing. The patient could not hold the tension required for symbolization. There was no space in which meaning could emerge—only equivalence, immediacy, and shame.

Symbolization, then, is not given—it is achieved. It depends on the capacity to tolerate emotional experience without collapsing into it. Where this capacity is absent, the mind operates through fusion and confusion. Where it begins to form, experience can be held, shaped, and eventually understood. Therapy becomes the place where this shift occurs—not by imposing meaning, but by allowing it to emerge.

DOI: 10.4324/9781003795803-14

## Jerome

Jerome liked certainty. He liked definitions. Sessions with him often felt like briefings: efficient, orderly, bracketed in terms such as emotional regulation and executive functioning. He had built his internal world the same way as his external one—structured, polished, and difficult to penetrate. His history—early parental loss, years of over-functioning, and a persistent sense of not quite belonging anywhere—rarely appeared in narrative form. It arrived instead in his need to make things make sense.

It took months before he brought in a dream. Even then, he qualified it before letting it land.

"It's nothing, really," he said, adjusting his cufflinks. "Just this recurring one. I'm in a courtroom, presenting a case. I know the material; I've done this before. But when I look down—my notes are gone. Just blank pages. I keep talking, but I know it's falling apart."

He paused.

"Anyway, it's probably just work stress. I've got two pitches this week."

I nodded but didn't follow him back into explanation. "What does it feel like, in the dream," I asked, "to be standing there without your notes?"

He shifted. His eyes flicked to the corner of the room.

"Exposed," he said eventually. Then: "Like I shouldn't be there."

I let the words hang, then said, "Maybe it's not about work. Maybe it's about what it's like when there's no script—no certainty. When you can't prepare your way through."

He didn't answer right away. His posture, usually upright and composed, gave slightly.

"Yeah," he said. "It's like... if I stop performing, I disappear."

Something shifted in that moment. The dream entered the room not as explanation, but as experience.

In the months that followed, more images appeared. A hallway with no doors. A voice that wouldn't carry. A gavel made of glass. A baby crying in a boardroom. He didn't always know how to describe them, and sometimes he laughed them off. But the part of him that once translated everything into language began to make room for what couldn't yet be named.

When I asked how he felt, he still reached for conceptual language—vulnerability, identity fragmentation, role ambiguity—but now he would add, "Or at least... something like that."

Symbolization hadn't replaced his intellect. It had softened its edges. The courtroom in his dreams was no longer something he had to master or explain, but something he could remain with. And for the first time, he wasn't trying to win the case. He was learning to listen to it.

## Two Configurations of Symbolic Emergence

Where Jerome required thought to loosen, Bill presented the opposite problem. He was not defended by language, but by its absence—by a kind of deadness where experience remained unformed. Here, symbolization did not emerge through insight, but under pressure. Something had to build, strain, and eventually give. What was required was not interpretation, but containment.

## Bill

By now, I knew how Bill carried tension—in his jaw, in the flatness of his voice, in the way he refused to linger on anything that might pull him inward. Sessions moved like heavy machinery: slow turns, friction, steel on steel. When we weren't circling the same terrain—broken pipes, incompetent coworkers, the price of car parts—we sat in a kind of psychic exhaust, thick with something unsaid.

The emotional content of the work rarely entered directly. It arrived sideways. A remark on his way out. A shift in timing. A dream, when it came, was usually dismissed before it landed. Still, they came.

"There's this garage," he said once. "Same one I used to work in with my dad. No windows. Heat everywhere. I'm trying to open the tool chest, but the drawers are jammed. Like the metal warped. I keep yanking on them. Then all at once they fall out. Tools spill everywhere. Only some of them don't look like tools. Some are bent. Some melted. Some sharp in a way they weren't supposed to be."

He paused.

"Anyway, probably just means I need to fix the latch."

The image held. The sealed air. The warped metal. The sudden collapse. Something had given under pressure.

I didn't interpret it. I let it remain.

Weeks later, he mentioned the garage again—this time with a memory. He'd smashed his hand there. Bled. His father told him to wipe it off and keep going. No crying.

The drawers—jammed shut. The tools—misshapen. The heat—unbearable.

He wasn't explaining the dream. He was entering it.

Over time, more fragments appeared. A locked door. A fire that didn't spread. A child inside a running car. The language stayed sparse, but the images accumulated. He still brushed them off, but not entirely.

"You'll probably want to talk about that," he said once, half-smirking. Then he waited.

He didn't decode the images. But he let them remain.

What had been sealed began to give.

## What It Asks of the Therapist

To develop the capacity to symbolize, the therapist has to stay with emotional material that arrives not as clarity but as density—as fragments, images, or tone. It is not about making the patient's world make sense, but about holding what does not yet.

With patients like Bill, symbolization arrives slowly, circuitously, and often against his will. His emotional life was buried under pragmatic debris: work stress, mechanical repairs, logistical complaints. To recognize symbol in this terrain, I had to attune more to pressure than to narrative—to the feel of an image rather than its meaning. Interpretation comes too soon and the drawer jams again. But when I stayed with the heat, the clutter, the fragments that did not yet cohere, something symbolic began to form—not as a solution, but as a tolerable encounter with inner life.

Jerome, by contrast, used clarity as a defense. He had language, but his dreams were treated as problems to solve, resolved too quickly to be lived. With him, I had to slow cognition—to create space for him to remain with the image rather than move past it. The courtroom dream—the moment he realized he had left his notes behind—marked an opening. His capacity to symbolize did not begin in insight, but in the pause. "Exposed," he said. The word held because it was not an idea—it was a feeling. With Jerome, the work required modeling what it meant not to know, to remain with the image long enough for meaning to take shape.

In both cases, the work required holding more than content—it meant staying with the disorientation of early symbolization. Murky images, displaced logic, abrupt resistance—all of it had to be allowed without correction. The task was to let the unconscious speak without rushing to translate, and to remain long enough for something to take form.

## Justification for the Placement of this Configuration

The *Capacity to Symbolize* follows *Tolerance of Frustration* within *Releasement Level A* because it depends on it. Without the ability to remain in the tension between desire and reality, experience cannot take symbolic form. It is either discharged, avoided, or distorted. Frustration tolerance creates the conditions in which something can be held long enough to be represented rather than expelled.

Only then can emotional experience begin to take shape as image, metaphor, or dream—no longer overwhelming or immediate, but capable of being reflected upon. Symbolization does not emerge through understanding alone, but through the capacity to stay with what has not yet been made sense of.

This shift also opens the next movement in the surrender process. As experience becomes representable, it can be encountered rather than defended against. The patient is no longer limited to reaction or evacuation but can begin to engage their inner world in a different way—one that allows deeper contact with what was previously unthinkable.

## Concluding Reflections

The capacity to symbolize reflects an expansion in the mind's ability to live with experience rather than evacuate it. When emotional life can take form—in image, language, or dream—the psyche gains space in which conflict, longing, and memory can be encountered without immediate discharge or distortion. Symbolization does not eliminate suffering; it renders it thinkable.

Within the surrender process, this capacity transforms raw affect into something that can be held in mind. What was once acted out, avoided, or collapsed into equivalence becomes available for reflection. In this way, symbolization establishes an inner field where psychic life can unfold rather than rupture.

The chapters that follow build on this capacity, tracing how the mind begins to take up its own experience more fully. Surrender deepens not through resignation, but through an increasing ability to remain present to inner life as it takes form.

# 12 The Capacity for Subjective Appropriation

The *Capacity for Subjective Appropriation* refers to the ability to recognize that one's experience—particularly what feels distressing or directed at others—is not merely happening to them but is being shaped from within. It involves a shift from experiencing thoughts, reactions, and conflicts as imposed or external, to recognizing them as arising from one's own inner world. This movement is not achieved through insight alone. It requires that the individual begin to feel these experiences as their own.

When this capacity develops, patients begin to recognize their experience as their own. What once felt imposed, confusing, or located in others can begin to be understood as arising from within. This shift allows for a different kind of engagement with inner conflict, one that makes deeper psychological work possible.

## Understanding Subjective Appropriation

Roussillon (2010) describes subjective appropriation as a process of emotional ownership, in which what has been projected, defended against, or disavowed is gradually recognized as part of the self. This is not simply a matter of understanding one's history or patterns, but of experiencing them as one's own.

Without this capacity, emotional life remains externalized. Inner conflict is located in others, experienced as intrusion, or kept at a distance through defensive organization. The individual may speak about themselves, but not from within themselves.

For some, this reflects a developmental absence. Without early experiences in which affect could be mirrored and metabolized, there is little internal space in which experience can be taken up. For others, the capacity exists but is defensively avoided. In these cases, turning inward does not bring coherence, but the threat of fragmentation. What might be appropriated is instead felt as overwhelming or annihilating.

These two configurations can be seen in Winston and Jerome. Winston's symbolic life is present, but his experience does not fully locate itself within him. What he feels, imagines, and attributes remains at the edges of

DOI: 10.4324/9781003795803-15

awareness, circulating without landing as his own. Jerome, by contrast, maintains access to feeling but organizes it through thought, keeping it at a distance. His difficulty is not access but allowing what arises—his reactions, meanings, and interpretations—to register without control as coming from him.

For psychic change to occur, the movement must shift from recognizing experience to taking it up. This includes not only what is felt, but what is projected, inferred, or located in others. Only when these can be recognized as one's own does integration become possible.

## Jerome

Jerome brought in repeated accounts of feeling subtly displaced by colleagues. The details changed, but the structure was familiar: someone interrupted, redirected, or took up an idea in a way that left him feeling diminished. He described these moments with precision, often reconstructing them almost argument by argument, as though accuracy itself might protect the experience from being altered.

In one session, after laying out such an exchange in careful detail, I said, "I wonder whether something in this experience feels familiar to you in a way that goes beyond this particular colleague."

He stiffened.

"I'm not sure why it always has to become something else," he said. "Sometimes what I'm describing is just what happened."

I did not press further. It felt important that he experience me as remaining with the event rather than trying to overtake it with meaning.

Several weeks later, he returned to a similar incident. Again, he had felt bypassed in a meeting, his contribution absorbed by someone else and returned without acknowledgment. This time, however, he paused while describing it.

"It was immediate," he said. "Before I had even thought about it, I knew what it was."

I asked, "You knew?"

He nodded. "I knew I was being minimized."

There was a silence.

Then he added, "At least that's how it landed."

The qualification was slight, but it marked something. For the first time, his certainty about the other gave way, however briefly, to an observation about the speed and force of his own experience.

Months later, a similar theme emerged again, but now with more inwardness. He had left a conversation at work feeling irritated and faintly humiliated. As he spoke, he began, as usual, by locating the problem in the other person's tone. Then he stopped.

"I can hear myself doing it," he said. "Fixing it there."

I waited.

He went on, more slowly. "It's not that they weren't dismissive. But the feeling is bigger than that. It gets there too fast."

I said, "Too fast for it to be only about this moment?"

He sat quietly for a while.

"Yes," he said. "I think so."

Even then, the recognition did not stabilize into full ownership. He would return to certainty, especially when feeling exposed. But something in the process had changed. What had previously been organized entirely as an external offense had begun, at moments, to be experienced as also arising from within. The work of appropriation did not happen in a single insight. It emerged gradually, through repeated encounters in which Jerome could begin to bear that his experience of others was shaped not only by what they did, but by what he brought to the encounter.

## Winston

By this point in the work, Winston's resistance had taken on a recognizable form. He rarely made accusations. He didn't lash out or challenge interpretations. What he resisted was not marked by intensity but by absence. Not silence, exactly. He could talk, and often did. But his speech had the weightlessness of a weather report: observations without affect, a voice trained to explain rather than to feel.

"I'm basically a good guy who got overwhelmed," he said once, in the same even tone he often used when speaking about his own life. "There's a kind of entropy to it now. Nothing acute. Just... erosion." It was the way physicians sometimes speak when they have learned to talk fluently about things they can no longer feel.

He talked about others—his housemates, his patients, the woman at the pharmacy—but without urgency or judgment. "She didn't fill my script," he said once. "I didn't correct her."

When I asked why, he shrugged. "Didn't seem worth it."

His stories had a way of circling events without ever quite landing inside them. It was difficult to locate a self within the telling.

Unlike Jerome, who projected tension outward with sharpness and suspicion, Winston dispersed his experience before it could fully gather. He didn't accuse me of anything; he just sometimes didn't show up. When he did, he would speak easily—but always just above the level of emotional contact. There was no friction, no edge—only a slow thinning out of presence, as though too much inwardness risked disorganization.

After one missed session, he returned and began speaking immediately, as though trying to refill the space he had vacated. I didn't interrupt. When there was a pause, I said, "You always make it easy to move past the gap. But I think sometimes the gap wants to be noticed."

He didn't respond, but his gaze stayed fixed on the floor. The next week, he showed up five minutes early.

I had begun to sense that his mildness was not benign. His quiet wasn't neutral; it was structured—a defense against being seen wanting. I never pressed too hard, but I didn't disappear either. Once, after a session in which he spoke almost the entire time about other people's problems, I said, "You tell stories like someone who's still standing outside them."

He paused, then nodded.

"Yeah," he said. "It's easier to care about other people."

That was the first moment something shifted.

Later, in a different session, he said, "I think I keep the place full, so I don't have to feel like it's me that's empty." He looked down, then added, "I'm not even sure I mean that. But it feels close."

I didn't answer right away.

He hadn't made a dramatic turn inward. But something in the diffusion had lessened. For a moment, he was no longer only describing the pattern from a distance. He was inside it, however briefly. What had long been dispersed around him had begun, almost imperceptibly, to gather around a self who could feel it.

## What It Asks of the Therapist

The *Capacity for Subjective Appropriation*—the process of recognizing one's projections as part of oneself—does not emerge through interpretation alone. It develops within a therapeutic process that can hold what has been projected without collapsing into it. For patients to claim what they have disowned, the therapist must offer a space that is both firm and unintrusive: a setting where meaning does not collapse the moment it emerges, and where discomfort can be held long enough to be recognized as one's own.

With Jerome, *Subjective Appropriation* was blocked by cognition. His insight ran ahead of his affect, creating a kind of pseudo-integration. He could name dynamics but not feel them. When what he located in others was reflected back too clearly, he deflected—intellectualizing, pathologizing, or accusing the therapist of siding with them. The work here required patience and a quiet resistance to taking the bait. What Jerome needed was not to be convinced but to be met—again and again—in the gap between knowing and feeling. His eventual shifts came not through confrontation, but through a slow unraveling of certainty.

Winston's difficulty, by contrast, was not in avoiding affect, but in lacking an internal structure to locate it. His resistance was organized around absence rather than defense. For him, the therapist's task was not to dismantle a fortress, but to help build a container. What he displaced was not hostile—it was diffused, disembodied. Here, the therapeutic presence had to be especially steady and quiet, offering an emotional contour where none yet existed.

*Subjective Appropriation* may begin at the edges—through dreams, discomfort, or insight—but it can only take root when transference becomes its living site. Without the enactment and containment of what has been externalized within the therapeutic relationship, appropriation risks staying intellectual. It is the transference that transforms it into something emotionally owned.

In both cases, the therapist's task is not simply to identify what has been disowned, but to hold the process by which it returns. This means resisting the urge to correct, to explain, or to push for ownership too soon. It also means trusting that, under the right conditions, what has been split off may find its way back—not as shame, but as recognition.

## Justification for the Placement of this Configuration

*Capacity for Subjective Appropriation* follows *Capacity to Symbolize* because symbolization alone does not guarantee ownership. Experience may take form, acquire meaning, and even become thinkable, while still feeling alien or externally caused. Subjective appropriation names the further movement by which what has been symbolized can also be recognized as one's own.

Roussillon (2010) emphasizes that psychic transformation requires not only representation, but appropriation: what has been projected, disavowed, or held at a distance must be taken up subjectively if it is to be integrated. Without this step, symbolized material can remain inert, alien, or defended against.

Its placement reflects its function as the movement from meaning into ownership, enabling patients to relinquish defensive detachment and participate more fully in their own experience. From here, surrender can deepen beyond recognition alone, because what has taken shape psychically can also begin to be lived as part of the self.

## Concluding Reflections

Subjective appropriation changes the status of experience. What was previously attributed, displaced, or recognized only at a distance begins to register as one's own. This does not happen all at once, and it does not happen through insight alone. It requires that the patient bear a different kind of nearness to inner life—one in which what had been organized in the other can no longer remain wholly there.

For Jerome, this meant loosening the certainty with which experience was located outside himself. For Winston, it meant allowing something long diffused and unclaimed to gather enough to be felt from within. In both cases, the movement was partial, fragile, and developmentally significant. The self was no longer only interpreting experience, or circling it, but beginning to inhabit it.

From here, surrender can deepen in a new way. Once experience is no longer merely symbolized but subjectively taken up, the patient is more able to remain with it without evacuating, explaining, or disowning it. What follows depends on that shift.

# 13 The Discipline Not to Reason

The *Discipline Not to Reason* is a crucial configuration in the process of surrender. It invites patients to encounter their inner worlds without immediately organizing them through rationalization or analysis. In this space, the compulsion to explain is suspended—not abandoned—so that raw, often nonverbal psychic material can be felt, metabolized, and gradually integrated.

This capacity for non-rational receptivity is essential to deeper surrender. Without it, the unconscious remains prematurely narrated—defended against through logic. With it, the psyche becomes porous, able to register experience in forms that are affective, sensory, imagistic—before words arrive.

## Understanding the Discipline Not to Reason

The *Discipline Not to Reason* draws on Bion's (1970) psychoanalytic use of Keats's notion of negative capability: the capacity to remain with uncertainty, emotional pressure, and emerging experience without rushing to impose coherence. The task is not to interpret too quickly, but to stay receptive—to allow what is still taking shape to register before it is organized.

Here, discipline is not rigidity but restraint. It does not mean rejecting thought, only postponing its organizing force. The aim is to let what is still emerging—image, feeling, tone, or association—appear before it is explained.

This is not a dismissal of intellect, but a reordering of sequence: first the image, then the insight; first the feeling, then the formulation. As Gendlin (1981) suggests, experience precedes language. Reason has its place—but not before the psyche has had time to speak in its own terms.

## Gabriella

By now, Gabriella could name her emotions in session—so long as they remained organized. She could link frustration to early caregiving, trace envy to past exclusions, account for sadness in terms that made sense. The

DOI: 10.4324/9781003795803-16

language was precise, the connections intact. And yet, something in her experience remained untouched.

One afternoon, she paused mid-sentence. "It's not that I don't feel," she said. "I just... prefer to understand it first." Her tone was even, but her hands were tightly clasped in her lap.

I didn't ask for clarification or expand the thought. "What happens if you don't?" I said.

She looked away. "Then it's just... there."

I didn't follow that immediately. The moment held.

After a pause, she added, more quietly, "And I don't know what to do with that."

In the sessions that followed, there were brief moments where the sequence loosened—feeling appearing before it could be accounted for, then receding again. Once, after describing a diffuse sense of emptiness, she stopped.

"It doesn't really make sense," she said. "There's nothing wrong."

I didn't move to organize it. The feeling remained, unanchored.

She shifted in her seat. "I don't like not knowing what it is."

"I know," I said.

She didn't elaborate further, but she didn't move away either.

The change was not in what she understood, but in what she could briefly remain with. The part of her that relied on explanation did not disappear, but it no longer closed the moment as quickly. At times, something could appear without being named, and persist for a few seconds longer before being taken up or pushed aside.

## Jerome

By this point in the work, Jerome no longer approached every session with the same immediate certainty. He had begun to notice how quickly he moved to organize experience—how reflexively he turned dreams, affects, and moments of destabilization into something named and manageable. But recognizing that tendency had not altered it. If anything, it made the pressure to get it right more immediate.

He came in one day with a dream he said had stayed with him all week. He described it carefully: he was back in a courtroom, but this time he was not speaking. Someone else was arguing the case, using his notes, his phrasing, even his voice. He sat at the table unable to interrupt.

"It's probably displacement," he said almost immediately. "Or envy. Or the usual control themes."

I said nothing.

He looked at me, waiting.

Finally he asked, "You're not going to say anything?"

"I'm trying to stay with the dream," I said.

He gave a faint, impatient smile. "Right."

But the smile didn't hold. He looked down at his hands.

After a while, he said, more quietly, "The strange part wasn't that someone else was speaking. It was that I knew the argument was wrong, and I still couldn't stop it."

The room grew still.

He might have moved into explanation there—he often did—but he didn't. The sentence seemed to leave him without footing.

I said, "You knew it was wrong."

He nodded.

"And couldn't interrupt."

Another nod.

He exhaled, but didn't speak.

"Helpless," he said finally. Then, after a pause: "No... not exactly."

He went quiet again.

I didn't ask him to clarify.

A few moments later, he said, "It was more like... I wasn't there anymore. The structure kept going, but I was out of it."

He didn't elaborate.

In another session, weeks later, he returned to the same dream without leading with an explanation.

"I keep thinking about that feeling," he said. "Not the dream exactly. Just that sense that something in me gets replaced the minute I try to understand it."

I said, "Replaced."

He nodded.

"That's what I'm starting to catch," he said. "I say something real, and then I can feel myself correcting it."

He stopped there.

"What happens if you don't?" I asked.

He gave a short laugh, but it didn't last. "Then it's unfinished."

We sat in that.

He shifted in his chair, then looked down again. "I don't usually leave things like that."

Another pause.

Then, more quietly: "But it's still there."

## What It Asks of the Therapist

To foster the discipline not to reason, the therapist must first sustain it within themselves. In both Gabriella's and Jerome's cases, meaning had to be suspended—not pursued too quickly. The work was not to name what was happening, but to remain with it as it emerged.

This requires tolerating the absence of immediate meaning and resisting the pull to organize experience prematurely. With Gabriella, this meant allowing silence to extend without filling it, even when she moved to restore order. With Jerome, it meant not following him into explanation, and allowing a dream or feeling to remain unformulated, even as he tried to define it.

Both patients were capable of insight. That was never the difficulty. What they required was a space in which experience could register before it was organized—where something could appear without being immediately taken up and explained.

Here, the therapist remains in contact with what has not yet taken shape, without resolving it. Insight may come, but only after something has first been allowed to exist without it.

## Justification for the Placement of this Configuration

The *Discipline Not to Reason* follows the *Capacity for Subjective Appropriation* in Releasement Level A, building on the patient's capacity to emotionally own their experience. In the *Capacity for Subjective Appropriation*, projections and defenses are taken up as aspects of the self. This makes possible a further demand: remaining with experience without immediately organizing it through thought.

Without this prior movement, the suspension of reasoning can become detachment rather than receptivity. When experience is not yet felt as one's own, the absence of interpretation does not deepen contact—it leaves the patient unanchored. Emotional ownership provides the grounding needed to tolerate ambiguity and uncertainty without withdrawing from the experience itself.

This configuration aligns with Bion's (1970) use of negative capability, in which both therapist and patient engage the analytic process without seeking immediate answers. Here, thinking is not abandoned, but deferred, allowing what has begun to emerge to unfold without premature organization.

## Concluding Reflections

The *Discipline Not to Reason* alters the sequence of experience. Thought no longer leads. What emerges is allowed to arrive before it is named, explained, or brought under control. For patients like Gabriella and Jerome, this does not mean the loss of thinking, but a restraint of it—the capacity to remain with what has not yet taken form, without moving to organize it.

In this state, experience is no longer immediately converted into meaning. It is encountered more directly, and therefore more fully. What had been organized too quickly can now be felt in its original intensity, without the usual protections of explanation or distance.

But this shift has consequences. As receptivity deepens, something else begins to stir: pain that can no longer be kept at bay. What happens when the act of surrender brings suffering to the surface? The next chapter takes us there.

# 14 The Suffering Necessary for Transformation

The *Discipline Not to Reason* loosens the hold of explanation, allowing affect to emerge without immediate understanding. In that suspension, something begins to press forward—experience that has not been fully formed, affect that has not been named, pain that has not been lived.

The *Suffering Necessary for Transformation* is the configuration in which that pain comes into view. No longer managed through explanation or projection, it must be experienced. The patient meets what has long been avoided: the ache of unmet need, the weight of past experience, the pressure of emotional truths that could not previously be borne. This is not suffering for its own sake, nor does it inherently produce growth. It is a threshold condition—one that makes transformation possible but does not guarantee it.

To avoid this suffering is to remain fixed. Intellectualization, retreat, or premature meaning-making may soften its impact, but they also interrupt the process. Turning toward the experience—remaining with it without disintegration—creates the conditions under which something new may take form. What could not be thought begins, gradually, to become thinkable.

## Understanding Suffering as a Catalyst for Transformation

Psychoanalytic thinking has long recognized that psychological growth depends on the capacity to bear emotional pain. For Wilfred Bion (1962, 1970), learning from experience is inseparable from tolerating what is initially overwhelming; without this, experience cannot be transformed into thought. Catastrophic change marks the point at which existing structures give way, making room for something not yet known.

Antonino Ferro (2006) describes how unprocessed experience, when it cannot be symbolized, circulates in repetitive patterns that organize the analytic field and limit the emergence of new meaning. When it can be borne, that repetition loosens and movement becomes possible.

For Melanie Klein (1946), this capacity is located in the depressive position, where guilt, loss, and ambivalence can be sustained without retreat into splitting. Donald Winnicott (1965) similarly emphasizes the necessity of

DOI: 10.4324/9781003795803-17

re-entering earlier experience and living it through, in the presence of another, for it to be transformed.

Across these perspectives, suffering does not lead neatly to growth. It marks a point of contact—something that cannot be bypassed, only endured. Whether it becomes transformative depends on whether it can be held, thought, and survived within the analytic relationship.

## Winston

Winston did not speak of suffering directly. It showed in how he arrived—slouched, faintly smelling of alcohol, his speech uneven, at times trailing off mid-sentence. He did not complain or assign blame. The impression was of something worn down over time, as if whatever once held him together had been giving way for years.

In the early phase of treatment, his material remained largely logistical: his schedule, his tenants, the condition of the house. When something more personal appeared, it did so obliquely—through small disruptions. A missed birthday. A voicemail he replayed but did not return. His tone remained flat, occasionally apologetic, but difficult to locate. What registered was not what he said, but what did not come through.

At one point, he mentioned his brother's funeral. "I didn't cry," he said. "Everyone else did. But I couldn't feel it. It was like I was watching it happen to someone else." I did not pursue it. The silence was allowed to stand.

After a pause, he added, "I think I started disappearing around then."

He looked down. "It was like... if I let myself feel it, I wouldn't come back."

He did not elaborate. The moment passed. But something had shifted—not in intensity, but in how close he came to it. These moments began to recur. He would stay with something a few seconds longer before drifting. At times, he seemed to register his own absence as it was happening, without interrupting it.

In another session, he described visiting his father in the hospital—his father, a surgeon, still exacting in manner. "I brought him one of those fruit bars he used to like. He didn't say thanks. Just looked at it and asked if I'd gained weight." He gave a brief laugh that did not quite land. "I think I wanted him to see me. Just once."

He continued without looking up. "I left it on the tray. He didn't touch it."

I said, after a moment, "You brought something to him."

Winston nodded, almost imperceptibly. After a few seconds, he added, "Yeah. I don't know why I thought it would be different." The room held the sense of something offered and not taken up.

## Jerome

Jerome often moved quickly past anything that threatened to slow him down. When something uncomfortable appeared, it was named, categorized, and set aside. In session, this took the form of efficiency—he reported, explained, concluded. There was little space for anything to linger.

One session marked a shift in that pattern. He described a humiliating interaction with a colleague, then dismissed it. "It's just part of the job," he said. "Politics."

The therapist did not follow the explanation.

"What was it like to be there?"

Jerome adjusted in his seat. "Fine," he said, then paused. "I mean—it was… awkward." Another pause. "Like I wasn't supposed to be there."

He looked away. "Like I got caught in something I didn't understand."

The room held.

Then, more quietly: "Like I was five again. Trying to convince my mother I hadn't broken the lamp."

He exhaled, almost immediately straightening. "Which is ridiculous," he added. "It's not the same thing."

But the shift had occurred. Not in what he said, but in how briefly he had let it come through.

In the weeks that followed, he returned to a recurring dream. A courtroom. No notes. No defense. A judge watching.

He had previously dismissed it—"performance anxiety." Now he described it differently.

"I'm talking, but I can't hear myself," he said. "The words are there, but… they don't land."

The therapist waited.

After a moment: "It's like I'm supposed to be convincing someone of something, but I don't know what it is."

He gave a short laugh. "Which doesn't make sense."

"What happens if it doesn't have to make sense?" the therapist asked.

He frowned. "Then what am I supposed to do with it?"

He didn't move away from the question, but he didn't settle into it either.

Over time, the dream did not resolve so much as shift. The courtroom gave way to other spaces—narrow hallways, locked bathrooms, rooms where his voice wouldn't carry. He spoke about them with less certainty, but also with increasing discomfort, as if something was being approached without a way to organize it.

At times, he would begin to follow one of these images, then interrupt himself. "There's probably an explanation," he would say, almost reflexively.

But the explanations came more slowly now.

In one session, after a long silence, he said, "I don't like this version of me."

He didn't specify which version.

A few minutes later, he added, "It feels like if I stop holding things together, there's nothing underneath that holds."

He looked up briefly, then away again.

The thought remained unfinished.

## What It Asks of the Therapist

In both cases, the work did not move forward through what the therapist said, but through what she could bear. Not the patient's behavior, but the feeling as it emerged—unstructured, uncontained. She did not move to organize it or bring it to clarity. She remained with it. That capacity—to stay without altering the moment—allowed something to take shape that had previously been avoided.

With Jerome, the task was to resist aligning with his need to make sense of things too quickly. His intellect did not need to be dismantled, but it could not be allowed to take precedence. When he moved to explain, the therapist stayed close to the point just before explanation—the place where something had registered but not yet been organized. The work depended on holding that interval without closing it.

With Winston, the difficulty was different. His suffering did not present directly; it appeared in its effects—missed sessions, disconnection, a kind of drift in the room. The pull was to compensate, to organize what he could not. The therapist had to resist that pull. She maintained the frame without filling in what was absent, allowing his experience to register in the room without being taken over.

In both cases, suffering was not treated as something to be resolved. It was approached as something that had to be undergone—without collapse, and without substitution. The therapist's role was not to lead the patient through it, but to remain where it became possible for the patient to stay.

## Justification for the Placement of this Configuration

The *Suffering Necessary for Transformation* follows the *Discipline Not to Reason* because without some loosening of explanation, the patient cannot remain with what emerges. The pull to make sense of things too quickly either organizes the experience before it is felt or pushes it out of reach entirely.

When suffering appears without that shift, it is not taken in. It is managed—explained, displaced, or moved past. What is required is not exposure, but the capacity to stay with what has not yet taken form.

The earlier work makes this possible. It creates enough space for something to register without being immediately resolved. In that space, suffering is no longer approached as something to be understood, but as something that must be undergone.

Only then does it begin to change. Not because it is interpreted, but because it is held long enough to take shape, until something in the patient's way of holding it can no longer be maintained.

## Concluding Reflections

Suffering is not the end of surrender. It constitutes a turning point. Here, the patient does not move past pain but allows it to register. For patients like Jerome and Winston, this meant letting sorrow, humiliation, or despair remain present without moving to correct or explain it. They begin to locate themselves within the experience rather than standing outside it.

This alters the ground of the work. As pain is faced more directly, the need for control—whether through perfection, explanation, or withdrawal—begins to loosen. Not by force, but through sustained contact: with the experience itself, with the therapist, and with what had previously remained unformulated.

The *Suffering Necessary for Transformation* is not a moment of catharsis. It is the capacity to bear what had previously been unendurable and to remain with it without splitting away from it. In that sense, suffering does not resolve. It becomes part of what can be held.

What begins as stillness does not remain contained. When pain is no longer managed or avoided, it takes form—sometimes as rupture, sometimes as grief, sometimes as expression not yet organized. In this way, suffering begins to give rise to what can follow. It is not a release from suffering, but a change in how it is lived.

# 15 Purification (Catharsis)

The *Purification* configuration resists precise clinical definition. It appears across Greek tragedy, mystical writing, and psychoanalytic theory, yet does not settle into a single form. The word 'catharsis', from the Greek *kathairein*, refers to cleansing or purging. In therapy, what is released is not sin, nor suffering itself, but what has remained unsaid—what could not be metabolized and had to be carried alone.

In ancient drama, catharsis marked a collective reckoning. The audience responded not only to Oedipus or Antigone, but to something shared. Through that recognition, tension gave way to a form of release.

In analytic work, the process is less visible but no less consequential. It does not erupt; it unfolds. It occurs when something previously unexpressed enters the room—not only as narrative, but as affect. Tears, silence, stillness, or regression may signal the same shift: a loosening of what had been held in place.

What gives this moment its significance is not the release alone, but that it occurs in the presence of another. As Wilfred Bion (1962) described in his theory of container and contained, the therapist's mind must function as a vessel capable of receiving the patient's fear, grief, or rage without becoming overwhelmed. This function is not passive. What is received is altered. The raw elements of experience—what Bion termed beta elements—are taken in, held, and gradually returned in forms that can be thought. In this sense, purification is not simply an unburdening. It marks a change in the patient's relation to what has already begun to be thought.

## Understanding Purification in Psychoanalysis

Sigmund Freud and Josef Breuer (2001) introduced the concept of catharsis through their early work on the talking cure. They observed that when patients gave expression to repressed, often traumatic, experiences, a form of relief could follow. But the effect did not lie in expression alone. It depended on the analytic frame—on the presence of another and the act of bringing into language what had been disavowed.

Catharsis, in analytic terms, is not ventilation. It is a psychic event that creates the possibility for reorganization. This is reflected in Ernst Kris's

DOI: 10.4324/9781003795803-18

(1952) concept of regression in the service of the ego, in which earlier affective states are re-entered not to relive them, but to allow what was previously unassimilated to be taken in.

Parallels appear in mystical traditions, where transformation is linked to a process of stripping away. St. John of the Cross (1959) described a "dark night" in which the self is emptied of familiar structures and identifications. What follows is not clarity, but a passage through disorientation. Change occurs not through understanding, but through what can no longer be maintained.

Similar themes appear in the work of Rumi and Hafiz (Lewis, 2000; Hafiz, 2010), where the self is depicted not as something to be protected, but as a place where experience arrives and is received. Their language differs from psychoanalysis, but the underlying movement is recognizable: what is endured, when held in the presence of another, can begin to take on form.

Within psychoanalysis, *Purification* is not a discrete event but a process that unfolds in the analytic relationship. It depends on the therapist's capacity to receive and transform affect the patient cannot yet hold. Here again, Bion's concept of alpha function (1962) is at work: unprocessed experience is taken in and rendered thinkable. This transformation is not intellectual. It occurs through a relational process that allows experience to become symbolized.

Through this work, previously repressed material is not only accessed but altered. It can be named, felt, and, over time, integrated. The result is not simply relief, but a closer relation to one's emotional life. What changes is not the existence of pain, but the capacity to remain in contact with it without being overtaken or cut off from it.

## Gabriella

As Gabriella's trust in me deepened, the changes were slight but noticeable. At times she would pause mid-sentence, as if unsure whether to continue, allowing something less controlled to enter before gathering herself again.

In one session, she began describing a memory from childhood—standing alone in the hallway while her parents argued behind a closed door. She spoke evenly at first, attending to the details. Then she stopped. The image seemed to hold.

After a moment, she said, more quietly, "I remember not knowing if anyone was coming out."

The shift was subtle. Her voice did not break, but something in it loosened. The distance she usually maintained from her experience was less intact.

I said, "It sounds like you were left there with something you had to hold on your own."

She looked up, her expression sharpening briefly, then softening. Her eyes filled, though she did not look away. The recognition did not expand into narrative. It remained where it was.

The moment passed without elaboration. But something had altered—not in intensity, but in contact. The memory was no longer only described. It had been entered, if only briefly, and in the presence of another.

In the sessions that followed, Gabriella referred back to the hallway more than once, each time with slightly less distance. She did not speak of release, nor did she frame the experience as relief. What changed was more contained: she could remain with the feeling longer without closing it down.

This was not a dramatic shift. Nothing was discharged or resolved. But something that had been held in isolation was now, in part, shared. That change—limited, partial, but real—marked a different relation to her own experience.

## Jerome

Jerome rarely stumbled over his words. His sentences, like his suits, were precise—structured, economical, and never without a point. In the early phases of treatment, he approached therapy as a place to think clearly, not to feel. He could recount painful experiences with fluency, arranging them into explanations that held together. It kept things ordered. It kept him intact.

In one session, he began describing a familiar memory.

"I must have been eight or nine," he said. "I'd done something—honestly, I don't even remember what—and they sent me to my room. It wasn't unusual."

He continued without hesitation. "I remember the light on the wall shifting. Late afternoon, I think. And I could hear them downstairs. Not clearly—just... movement. Voices, but not distinct."

He paused briefly, then added, "I remember thinking the door might not open. Not in a dramatic way. Just... it didn't seem certain that it would."

He spoke evenly, as he often did, but something in the rhythm of his speech had begun to change. The sentences no longer followed with the same precision. He paused, then restarted, as if the sequence no longer held as cleanly.

I said, "You're describing it very clearly. But something about it doesn't seem settled."

He looked at me, briefly disoriented. "I don't know what you mean," he said, though without his usual certainty.

There was a longer pause than usual. He shifted in his seat, then said, more quietly, "I can't quite get it to—" He stopped, then tried again. "It's not organizing the way it usually does."

He stopped again.

The room became still. He did not move to clarify or reinterpret what he had just said. For a moment, he seemed unable to.

His eyes filled, though he did not immediately respond to it. He remained where he was, without turning back to explanation. The effort to regain composure was visible, but he did not complete it.

He paused, then resumed, though without his usual precision. The thread had shifted, and he did not fully recover it.

What stood out was not the emergence of feeling alone, but the interruption of his usual way of holding it. He did not resolve the experience or restore coherence. He remained in a state he could not fully organize.

In the following sessions, he returned to the memory, but less as an account to be understood and more as something that did not yet make sense to him.

"I keep thinking I should be able to explain it," he said once. "But it doesn't... reduce."

He referred to the session as "losing the thread," though he did not frame it as relief.

Nothing was discharged. Nothing was resolved. But something in his way of maintaining himself had been disrupted. He could no longer rely entirely on the structures that had previously kept experience contained.

## What It Asks of the Therapist

For *Purification* to occur, the therapist offers more than presence. They maintain a position in which what has been held out of awareness can begin to enter without being organized too quickly. This moment cannot be produced. It emerges when the patient's usual way of managing experience no longer holds, and something less structured comes forward. The task is to remain with it without moving to clarify or contain it prematurely.

With Gabriella, this required close attention to shifts that were easy to miss. What mattered was not what she said, but where she paused, and whether she could remain there. When feeling began to register more directly, the work was not to interpret it, but to stay with her as she experienced it without immediately closing it down. The change was not dramatic. It was that she did not have to hold it entirely on her own.

With Jerome, the task was different. His difficulty was not access to experience, but his need to organize it. When that capacity faltered, the impulse to restore coherence was immediate. The therapist's role was not to challenge his defenses directly, but to recognize the moment when they no longer functioned and to avoid stepping in to reestablish them. What mattered was that the disruption could remain in place long enough to be experienced, without being resolved.

This configuration requires the therapist to tolerate states that are not yet thinkable without moving to make them so too quickly. The pressure to interpret, reassure, or give shape to the experience can interrupt what is beginning to emerge. Containment here is not passive but involves maintaining contact without imposing structure.

As Wilfred Bion (1962) described, the therapist's capacity to receive and hold what the patient cannot yet think is central here. This function is at work without being made explicit. What cannot yet be organized is allowed to remain, rather than being shaped too quickly into meaning.

*Purification*, in this sense, is not defined by release. It depends on whether what emerges can be experienced in the presence of another without being withdrawn or reorganized prematurely. What changes is not simply that something is expressed, but that it is no longer held in isolation.

## Justification for the Placement of this Configuration

Purification rests on the capacity developed in the *Suffering Necessary for Transformation*. Until the patient can turn toward suffering without moving away from it—through explanation, dissociation, or other forms of control—what emerges here cannot be sustained.

In the *Suffering Necessary for Transformation*, the patient begins to remain with what had previously been avoided. In *Purification*, that contact deepens. What has been approached begins to take on a different form—not as insight, but as experience that is no longer held at a distance.

Premature contact with this configuration evokes retreat or a return to earlier forms of organization. What emerges exerts pressure on the patient's usual modes of managing experience. Without sufficient capacity to remain present, that pressure fails to be tolerated.

From a psychoanalytic perspective, catharsis is not an initiating event but a consequence. It becomes possible only after the patient can remain in contact with what has been previously unendurable. In this sense, purification does not introduce something new. It alters the patient's relation to what has already been encountered, allowing it to be experienced without immediate reorganization.

## Concluding Reflections

*Purification* constitutes a turning point, not an end. Pain does not resolve here. It takes form differently — no longer held entirely at a distance, but not yet fully organized.

For patients like Gabriella and Jerome, this did not take the form of dramatic release. For Gabriella, it meant remaining with feeling slightly longer than before, without closing it down. For Jerome, it meant moments in which his usual capacity to organize experience no longer held. In each case, what changed was not the presence of pain, but the way it could be experienced.

What makes this configuration possible is not the intensity of what emerges, but whether it can be sustained in the presence of another. Without that, the experience is avoided or reorganized too quickly. Within it, something remains in contact long enough to take on a different form.

As this occurs, the patient's relation to their internal world changes. Experience that had been kept separate can be approached with less immediate control or withdrawal. It does not resolve, but allows for sustained contact with what had previously been excluded.

*Purification* is not a discrete event, nor does it function as a clearing. It constitutes a point at which previous ways of holding experience no longer hold. That change—partial, uneven, but sustained—opens the possibility for further development.

# 16 Preparation for Love

*Preparation for Love* does not announce itself as love. It appears more quietly—as a change in what the patient can remain in contact with. Longing that would have been dismissed is allowed to register. Dependency, once warded off or managed, begins to surface in less mediated ways. The question is no longer whether these states exist, but whether they can be tolerated without immediate retreat.

What shifts here is not insight, but proximity. The patient begins to stay with experiences—wanting, missing, needing—that previously required distance. Ferro (2017) notes that painful emotional states, when held within the analytic setting, can become the basis for new forms of experience. At this point in the work, those states are no longer avoided as quickly. They are not yet organized, but they are no longer entirely disowned.

This brings the patient into contact with a familiar but difficult configuration: the coexistence of opposing feelings toward the same object. Klein (1946) described this as a developmental achievement—the capacity to hold love and aggression together without splitting. Here, that tension reappears in a more conscious form. The therapist may be experienced as needed and resisted, trusted and doubted. What matters is not resolving that tension but remaining in contact with it. From within that contact, something resembling the conditions for love begins to take shape.

## Understanding Preparation for Love

Klein's developmental model (1946) situates the capacity for love in the integration of early relational experience. The infant moves between satisfaction and frustration, attachment and anger. Over time, these experiences are no longer kept apart. The same object can be both loved and hated, depended on and resented. This integration does not eliminate conflict. It makes it tolerable.

*Preparation for Love* revisits this configuration. The patient is no longer organizing experience through clear divisions—idealized or devalued, self-sufficient or dependent—but encountering mixed states that cannot be easily resolved. The difficulty is not understanding these states but remaining in contact with them without restoring distance.

DOI: 10.4324/9781003795803-19

Anzieu's concept of the skin-ego (1989) offers another way of approaching this shift. The sense of having an internal boundary—something that can hold experience without immediate overflow—becomes central here. Without it, closeness threatens to overwhelm. With it, the patient can move toward and away from connection without losing coherence. The issue is not simply proximity to another, but whether that proximity can be registered internally.

A similar movement appears in spiritual writing, though described differently. St. John of the Cross (1959) and later Thomas Moore (2004) both describe a period in which familiar forms of comfort fall away. What remains is a more direct encounter with longing—without immediate relief or resolution. In clinical terms, this can be understood as a reduction in defensive organization. What had been managed or avoided becomes more available, but not yet transformed.

*Preparation for Love* is not a pause before something begins. It is a period in which the patient's relation to need, absence, and dependency is altered. Nothing is resolved here. But something becomes possible that was not possible before: remaining in contact with desire without immediately moving to defend against it.

## Winston

Winston continued to come each week, often arriving a few minutes late, settling into the chair with a quiet "Sorry," as if his presence required justification. He spoke easily about his schedule—patients, overnight calls, small repairs around the house—but when the conversation moved toward anything relational, it thinned.

"I don't really think about that stuff," he said once. "People wanting things from each other." A pause. "I think I missed that part."

He said it lightly, but then went quiet, as if something in the statement had gone further than he intended.

In another session, he described a dream.

"I was lying on a couch," he said. "Not mine. Somewhere else. And someone came in—just to check if I was still there." He shrugged. "They didn't say much. Just sat down."

I waited.

After a moment, he added, "It wasn't… uncomfortable."

He didn't elaborate. But he didn't move away from it either.

There were small moments like this that began to accumulate. He mentioned, almost in passing, watching an elderly couple outside a café.

"He helped her with her coat," Winston said. "Nothing dramatic. Just… stayed with her while she figured out the sleeve." He gave a brief exhale, something close to a laugh. "I don't know why that stuck with me."

I said, "You noticed the staying."

He nodded, though his eyes had shifted away.

At times, he would approach something more directly, then pull back just as quickly.

"I've set things up so it's simple," he said one afternoon. "No one really relies on me for anything emotional." A pause. "And I don't have to rely on anyone either."

He looked at me then, as if checking whether that would be understood as a strength.

I didn't answer right away.

After a few seconds, he added, more quietly, "It works."

But he didn't move on.

The change was not dramatic. It appeared in how long he could remain with something before reorganizing. Where he might once have deflected or flattened the moment, he began, at times, to stay.

In one session, he trailed off mid-sentence and looked down.

I said, "Something just came up."

He shook his head slightly. "It's nothing."

We sat there for a moment.

Then he said, without looking up, "Sometimes I think... it would be easier if someone just knew." A pause. "Without me having to explain it."

He stopped there.

He didn't withdraw from the statement, but he didn't develop it either. The wish appeared, briefly, without being organized or defended.

Over time, he began to recognize these moments as they were happening.

"I notice it sometimes," he said. "Like... wanting something and then trying to shut it down before it gets anywhere."

I asked, "And today?"

He considered that.

"I didn't shut it down as fast."

He said it without emphasis, but it stayed in the room.

For Winston, this was the work. Not forming a relationship, not articulating a clear desire, but remaining in contact with the emergence of need without immediately erasing it. The longing did not yet have direction. It appeared in fragments—through a dream, an image, a sentence that stopped halfway.

What changed was not its intensity, but its duration. It lasted slightly longer. It registered.

And he did not always move away.

## Bill

Bill usually started by talking about whatever had happened that week—work, something that broke around the house, traffic. He spoke in short stretches, then stopped, as if that was enough.

"I don't really do all that," he said once, when the conversation drifted toward relationships. He made a vague gesture with his hand. "Talking about feelings. Never saw the point."

I didn't respond.

He added, after a second, "Doesn't usually go well."

He drank most nights. Not something he emphasized—just mentioned it the way he mentioned everything else.

"Takes the edge off," he said. "Otherwise, things just... sit there."

"What sits there?"

He shrugged. "Stuff."

In one session, he described his wife telling him about a possible promotion.

"She was excited," he said. "Telling me all the details." A pause. "I didn't say much."

"What was happening for you?"

He looked off to the side. "I don't know. Just... felt far away all of a sudden." He frowned slightly. "Like I was supposed to feel something and didn't."

He didn't elaborate, but he didn't dismiss it either.

At other times, something else came through, less defended.

He talked about a dog he had as a kid.

"Used to wait for me by the door every day," he said. "Didn't matter what kind of day I had." A brief pause. "Just knew I was coming back."

He stopped there, but the tone had shifted—less certain.

Another time, he mentioned his grandmother.

"She'd leave the porch light on if she knew I was coming over late." He gave a small shrug. "Didn't say much. Just... left it on."

I said, "You remember that."

He nodded but didn't look up.

When I asked what he wanted now, he answered quickly.

"Nothing complicated. Quiet. Someone who doesn't need a whole lot."

A pause.

Then, almost as an afterthought, "Or someone I don't have to brace myself around all the time."

He seemed to register what he'd said only after it was out.

I said, "Not having to stay on guard."

He gave a short exhale. "Yeah."

He didn't expand on it. But he stayed with it longer than he usually would have.

Bill didn't move toward connection directly. When something close to it appeared, he minimized it, flattened it, or turned away. But it didn't disappear completely.

What changed was that it began to show up more often—and he didn't always shut it down right away.

"I catch it sometimes," he said in one session. "Thinking it'd be easier if I didn't have to be on edge all the time around people."

He shook his head slightly. "Then I just drop it."

I asked, "Today?"

He paused.

"Didn't drop it as fast."

For Bill, this was as far as it went. The want was there, but it stayed partial—appearing, then receding. He did not move toward it, but he was no longer entirely outside of it.

And at times, he let it remain, briefly, without covering it over.

## What It Asks of the Therapist

The therapist's task is not to draw out longing, but to avoid closing it down. What begins to appear is often brief and easily lost — a remark that goes slightly further than intended, a pause that is not immediately filled, a change in tone that signals something less defended.

The work is to notice these moments without enlarging them too quickly.

With Winston, this meant allowing his emerging wish for contact to remain only partially formed. When he spoke about someone sitting beside him in a dream, or noticed a couple lingering together, the therapist did not name this as longing or interpret it as desire. To do so would have outpaced him. Instead, she stayed close to what was already there, marking it lightly when needed and otherwise leaving it undisturbed.

With Bill, the task was different. His movement toward connection appeared as a reduction in bracing—within the room as well as beyond it—rather than the emergence of articulated want. When he spoke about not wanting things to "turn into something" or noticing that he hadn't "dropped it as fast," the therapist did not press for elaboration or reframe this as vulnerability. She remained alongside the moment without increasing its intensity.

In both cases, the therapist's role was to maintain a level of contact the patient could tolerate—not to deepen it prematurely, and not to withdraw from it. The work turns on pacing—staying within range of the patient's capacity to remain present.

These changes are easy to miss. They do not announce themselves. They appear as slight extensions of contact that may not repeat in the next session. The therapist registers them without relying on them.

A form of restraint is required—not neutrality as absence, but the capacity to remain engaged without shaping the moment too quickly. The therapist does not require the patient to clarify, expand, or stabilize what has just begun to emerge.

Over time, something changes: the patient can remain in contact with a wish, however faint, without immediately reorganizing around it.

## Justification for the Placement of this Configuration

*Preparation for Love* follows *Purification* because it depends on what has already shifted in the patient's relation to experience. After *Purification*, something that had been held out of contact is no longer entirely excluded. What changes here is not the emergence of new material, but the way existing experience can be tolerated.

This does not involve further release. It involves remaining with what has already come into contact, without moving to resolve or manage it prematurely.

If it were placed earlier, the patient would not yet be able to stay with these states. What appears here—wanting, missing, the beginning of dependency—would either be dismissed or reorganized into something more controlled. The work of purification makes it possible for these states to register at all. *Preparation for Love* tests whether they can remain.

From a psychoanalytic perspective, this is not a shift in content but in organization. The patient is no longer structured entirely around avoidance of certain affective states. Those states can now appear, but only briefly and often without coherence.

Winston's experience of wanting contact, and Bill's recognition of reduced defensiveness, both illustrate this. Neither represents a stable change. What is new is that these experiences are not immediately eliminated.

This does not introduce connection. The patient's relation to it alters. What had been managed or avoided can now be approached, but only within a limited range.

Placing it here reflects that sequence. The patient has already encountered what was previously excluded. The question now is whether they can remain in contact with it, even briefly.

## Conclusion

*Preparation for Love* does not bring resolution or a stable sense of connection. Certain experiences—wanting, missing, the presence of another—can be registered without immediate avoidance.

These moments are brief and inconsistent. They do not accumulate into a clear direction. What had to be avoided can appear, without immediate reorganization.

The tension between autonomy and dependency does not resolve. It can be borne without eliminating one side of it.

*Preparation for Love* is not a movement into relationship, but a change in what can be held in experience. What had to be excluded can enter experience, however briefly.

That is what makes further development possible.

# Part III
# Releasement Level B

## Transformational Surrender

The Neural and Affective Repatterning Systems

*Releasement Level B* reflects a change in how transformation is encountered. In *Level A*, the work involved coming into contact with experience that had been avoided or held at a distance. Here, the emphasis is less on contact and more on reorganization. The patient is no longer working toward something in the same way. Instead, changes may be observed that are not directly initiated or controlled.

This is not regression or collapse. The patient remains present, but the organization of experience begins to shift. States that were previously difficult to tolerate may now be remained with for longer periods, without immediate avoidance or restructuring. What shifts is not the content of experience, but the patient's relation to it.

The configurations that follow—*Non-Willing, Emergent Relationship, Ecstasy, Doubt, Contemplation,* and *Foreboding*—do not function as achievements. They arise within the process, often briefly and not repeatable on demand, and do not appear in a fixed sequence. Each reflects a moment in which experience is no longer organized in the usual way.

These shifts are not produced through effort. They occur outside of deliberate control, often in the context of sustained therapeutic work. When they appear, they are registered less as insight than as a change in orientation. The patient may notice a different way of being in relation to thought, feeling, or the presence of another, without being able to account for it.

From a neurobiological perspective, these changes can be understood as involving neuroplastic processes. Repeated experiences of remaining with affect within a stable relational context are associated with alterations in patterns of response over time. Systems involved in threat detection and habitual defense (including regions such as the amygdala and dorsal anterior cingulate) may become less dominant in certain contexts, while those associated with regulation, flexibility, and relational engagement may become more available.

DOI: 10.4324/9781003795803-20

This does not occur through intention alone. It is associated with repeated exposure to states that were previously avoided, in conditions that allow them to be experienced without overwhelming the system. Over time, these changes may be experienced less as effortful adaptation and more as a shift in how experience organizes itself.

These moments are often unstable. They may not persist and may not be recognized immediately. But they indicate that change is no longer occurring only at the level of insight or symbolic understanding. It is taking place within the organization of experience itself.

# 17 Non-Willing

In the progression of surrender, non-willing reflects a shift in how the patient relates to effort and control. It does not take the form of resignation or deliberate acceptance. Rather, it appears as a reduction in the need to organize experience through intention. The patient is no longer directing themselves toward a particular outcome, including the outcome of surrender itself.

This is not the absence of agency, but a change in its use. The impulse to shape, interpret, or resolve experience becomes less immediate. At times, the patient may remain with what is occurring without moving to act on it or make sense of it.

There is a difference between not knowing and no longer needing to resolve not knowing.

Non-willing cannot be produced deliberately. It appears when the patient is no longer organizing experience around goals, even implicitly. Thought does not disappear, but its urgency lessens. The patient may notice a capacity to remain with experience without immediately interpreting or redirecting it.

This condition echoes the writings of both mystics and psychoanalysts. As Meister Eckhart describes, "The man who has reached the highest stage… does not will God's will, or will to have no will. He is simply will-less; he lives outside the sphere of willing altogether" (Caputo, 1978, p. 176).

What this names clinically is a state in which experience is no longer organized around outcome, effort, or control. The patient is not trying to arrive anywhere—not even at surrender. Something is allowed to occur without being directed.

Bion (1970/2014) refers to an analytic position in which the analyst refrains from organizing what is not yet formed, allowing experience to unfold before it is shaped into meaning. This involves a capacity to remain with what is occurring without directing it toward resolution. In such moments, both patient and therapist may find themselves less oriented toward producing understanding and more able to stay with what is emerging as it is.

Non-willing, in this sense, is not disengagement. The patient remains present, but without the same pressure to direct or stabilize what is

DOI: 10.4324/9781003795803-21

occurring. These moments are often brief and may pass without being fully recognized. Yet they mark a change in the rhythm of experience: a temporary reduction in effort, in which something can unfold without being immediately shaped.

What follows are instances of this shift—moments in which direction gives way, however briefly, to a different form of presence.

## Jerome

"I've been thinking about last session," Jerome said as he sat down. "I realized I was probably avoiding something when I brought up the dream. It connects to the same pattern I mentioned before—the need to stay in control when things feel uncertain."

He paused, then continued.

"The dream itself wasn't that complicated. I was in a house I didn't recognize. There were people there, but I couldn't see them clearly. I think that's probably

about—"

He stopped.

"Actually, I'm not sure what it's about. I mean, it's probably about uncertainty. That would make sense."

I said nothing.

He went on, but more slowly.

"I guess I keep trying to get ahead of it. Like if I can explain it fast enough, it won't... turn into something else."

I said, "What happens if you don't?"

He didn't answer.

"I don't know... what I'm feeling."

I didn't respond.

After a moment, he began again.

"There's this memory—I don't know why this is coming up. It's nothing, really. Just... the corner of the kitchen table. My mother was in the other room. I think she was—"

He stopped. Looked down. Took a breath.

"I should be able to say this."

He tried again, then let it go.

"I don't know what that was."

I said, "Okay."

He didn't continue.

He stayed there.

I didn't speak.

After a while, he glanced toward the window.

"The light's changing," he said.

I nodded.

He looked back down.

He shifted in his chair and let out a breath.
"It feels... different," he said.
He didn't return to the memory.

## Gabriella

Gabriella spoke carefully, as she often did, keeping her tone measured. "I was thinking about something from when I was little," she said. "I was in my room. I had a doll—I don't remember where it came from."

She paused.

"I remember wanting to be held," she said. Then, quickly, "But I knew better than that."

I didn't respond.

She sat with it for a moment, then added, "It didn't make sense to want that. It wasn't... how things were."

Her voice trailed off.

She didn't move to explain it further. Didn't qualify it. Didn't shift away.

The room remained as it was.

After a while, she said, more quietly, "I can still feel that. A little."

I nodded.

She looked down at her hands. "It's strange," she said. "I would usually have told myself not to think about it."

She didn't say anything else.

The feeling didn't disappear, but she didn't push it away either.

After some time, she let out a small breath.

"It's not as bad as I thought," she said.

She didn't elaborate.

## What It Asks of the Therapist

In these moments, the therapist's task is not to move the process forward, but to refrain from doing so.

The impulse to ask, clarify, or make sense becomes more noticeable. The patient pauses, something begins to form, and the pressure to help it along—to name it or bring it into coherence—can be strong. In *Non-Willing*, that impulse is held back.

The therapist remains present, attentive, and responsive, without directing the moment toward meaning or resolution. What is emerging is allowed to remain before it has taken shape.

With Jerome, this meant not responding to his halted speech with questions or interpretation. The silence was not filled. Nothing was added. The moment was allowed to remain incomplete.

With Gabriella, the therapist did not move to reframe or soften the memory she described. Her longing was neither questioned nor elaborated. It was not turned into something more manageable or more understandable.

In both cases, the therapist's role was to not intervene prematurely. The work was to remain with the patient without organizing the experience for them.

This position can be difficult to sustain. It requires tolerating the absence of movement, the absence of clarity, and the possibility that nothing will come of the moment. It also requires setting aside the expectation that the session should lead somewhere.

*Non-Willing* in the patient is supported by a similar restraint in the therapist: a willingness to remain present without directing what occurs.

## Justification for the Placement of this Configuration

*Non-Willing,* situated within *Releasement – Level B,* arises only after foundational capacities have been established and the patient has begun to loosen their orientation toward outcome.

In earlier configurations—particularly *Preparation for Love*—openness and longing can be present but remain organized around expectation. The wish is still directed—toward being understood, received, or relieved.

*Non-Willing* begins when that orientation weakens. The patient no longer engages the work in order to obtain something. The effort to move the process forward—subtle as it may be—drops away.

This is not collapse and it is not transcendence. The patient remains present, but without organizing their experience toward gain or resolution.

In this sense, *Non-Willing* marks a threshold. It is not a development of new capacity, but a loosening of what has been guiding the process. Without this shift, the work remains shaped by intention.

*Emergent Relationship* depends on this loosening. If the work is approached with direction or expectation, what follows remains structured by that effort. *Non-Willing* creates the conditions in which something relational can arise without being shaped in advance.

It is not an achievement, but a relinquishment that allows further development.

## Conclusion

*Non-Willing* is marked by a change in how the patient relates to the process. The need to move forward, to understand, or to arrive at something begins to recede.

What replaces it is not clarity but the absence of pressure to produce it.

The patient may still speak, reflect, or feel, but these are no longer organized toward an outcome. There is less urgency to resolve what is happening, and less effort to shape it into something coherent.

In the room, this often appears as a pause that is not corrected, a feeling that is not explained, or a moment that is allowed to remain incomplete.

The therapist's role is to remain with the patient in that state without organizing it for them. This requires tolerating the absence of movement and setting aside the expectation that the session should lead somewhere.

What follows from this position cannot be produced directly. It depends on the patient's willingness to remain without directing their own experience.

*Non-Willing* alters the conditions under which the work proceeds. From this position, something relational may begin to take shape—without being sought or guided.

# 18 Emergent Relationship

*Emergent Relationship* begins as contact between patient and therapist changes. The interaction is less organized by effort—less shaped by what the patient is trying to achieve, avoid, or understand.

At first, it can be hard to locate. The patient may speak without tracking the therapist as closely. A thought is offered without being adjusted. A moment is allowed to remain incomplete. The therapist is no longer approached in the same way—not read as carefully, not managed as deliberately.

At the same time, something shifts in how the patient is with their own experience. What arises is not immediately organized, explained, or corrected. It is allowed to remain as it is.

Nothing new is being introduced. What becomes noticeable is the absence of what had been structuring both the exchange and the patient's relation to what they are experiencing.

Earlier in the work, even openness carries direction. The patient may want to be known, to be understood, or to arrive at something. That orientation begins to fall away. What is said—and what is felt—is no longer guided in the same way.

This does not make the relationship more intense or more expressive. It becomes less structured. The patient may still hesitate or withdraw, but these movements are no longer governed by the same effort to control how the moment unfolds.

These moments are easy to miss. A statement isn't revised. A silence isn't filled. A response isn't shaped to manage the therapist. A feeling is not immediately turned into something else. What distinguishes them is not their content, but the absence of effort organizing them.

The cases that follow show how this form of contact begins to appear in the room.

## Bill

By this point in the work, Bill's sessions had begun to change, though not in a way he would have named.

DOI: 10.4324/9781003795803-22

He still spoke about practical things—repairs, routines, the structure of his days—but there were moments when he didn't move through them in the same way. He would pause, not to organize what he was saying, but because something had interrupted the usual flow.

In one session, he was describing time spent in his garage.

"I sit out there sometimes," he said. "Not doing anything. Just sitting."

He glanced up briefly, then back down.

"I think I miss myself sometimes," he added. "Like I'm waiting for me to come back."

He didn't elaborate.

The moment held. He didn't move away from it or try to make it clearer.

After a few seconds, he let out a small breath.

"It's not a bad feeling," he said. "Just... different."

He didn't look toward me to see how I would take it.

In earlier sessions, he would have filled the space—offered a joke, returned to something concrete, or rephrased what he meant. Here, he didn't. The thought remained as it was.

Over time, these moments appeared more often. He would say something and leave it without adjusting it. A silence would settle and remain. He began to speak without organizing his words around how they might be received.

Nothing in his presentation became more expressive or more resolved. But the way he occupied the room changed. There was less effort to manage what was happening—both in what he said and in how he stayed with it.

## Winston

Winston had spent years taking care of other people while letting his own life drift into disrepair. He spoke about it without much emphasis—patients, people staying in his house, things getting out of hand—but never in a way that suggested he intended to change it.

In sessions, he moved quickly. He filled space, circled ideas, made sharp observations about himself that didn't seem to land anywhere. If something edged too close, he would shift—into humor, into detail, into something else.

One afternoon, he was talking about a man he'd let stay with him—someone who hadn't paid rent in months.

"I don't even like him," Winston said. "He eats my food, doesn't clean, barely says thank you."

He gave a short laugh.

"I don't know why I let this happen."

He went quiet.

Normally, he would have kept going—explained it, justified it, or moved on. This time, he didn't.

He looked off to the side, then down at his hands.

"It's not even about him," he said after a moment. "It's just... familiar."

He didn't elaborate.

The silence held. He didn't move to fill it.

After a few seconds, he exhaled.

"I don't know what that is," he added. "But it's there."

He didn't look toward me to see how I would take it.

In earlier sessions, he would have turned the moment into something sharper—an interpretation, a criticism, something he could control. Here, he left it as it was.

Over time, these moments began to appear more often. He would say something and not follow it with explanation. A pause would settle and remain. He no longer seemed to organize what he said around how it might be received.

Nothing in him became more stable or more resolved. But the way he occupied the room changed. There was less effort to direct what was happening—less movement away from what he had already said.

## What it Asks of the Therapist

In these moments, the therapist's role changes in a subtle but decisive way. The work is not to help the patient understand or articulate their experience, but to refrain from interfering with how it unfolds.

The therapist functions less as an active container and more as a presence that does not intrude or reshape what is forming. The emphasis is not on holding in the traditional sense, but on not altering the patient's emerging contact with their own experience.

This requires a particular discipline. The therapist must resist the impulse to clarify, affirm, or extend what the patient has said. When Bill remarks that he misses himself, or when Winston leaves a statement without explaining it, the moment does not need to be developed. It needs to be left intact.

The pressure to respond can be strong in these moments—especially as something more genuine begins to appear in the room. But responding too quickly reinstates the old structure: experience followed by organization. That sequence loosens.

This reintroduction of structure does not always take an obvious form. It may appear as a minimal acknowledgment, a slight shift in tone, or a question that seems to follow the patient's lead but subtly redirects it. Even the wish to remain aligned with the patient can become a form of interference if it organizes what is still in the process of taking shape. What is required here is not neutrality in a technical sense but a restraint in relation to one's own participation. The therapist must recognize the point at which response becomes organization and allow the moment to remain where it is, even when it feels incomplete or unconfirmed.

At the same time, the transference is undergoing a change in its organizing function. The patient's experience is no longer structured to the same degree around anticipation of the therapist's response or the need to manage how it will be received. The other remains present but is less actively organized against or oriented toward. This places a corresponding demand on the therapist: not to re-establish themselves as the central point around which experience must be shaped, even implicitly. The task is not to withdraw but to remain present in a way that does not require the patient to organize themselves in relation to that presence.

Countertransference often shifts as well. The therapist may notice a reduction in urgency—less pressure to interpret, less need to move the session forward. There may be a sense of steadiness, or even a mild pull toward involvement as the patient becomes less defended. These responses are useful only insofar as they are not acted upon prematurely.

The task is simple, but exacting: to remain present without shaping what is emerging.

## Justification for the Placement of this Configuration

*Emergent Relationship* follows *Non-Willing* because it depends on a prior shift: the reduction of effortful engagement with experience.

In *Non-Willing,* the patient relinquishes the attempt to direct, solve, or make use of what arises. Experience is no longer organized toward an outcome. Without this, what appears is quickly drawn back into interpretation or control.

Here, something different begins to occur. The patient does not move away from what they have said, but they also do not elaborate it. The experience is allowed to stand without being developed.

This marks a change in position. The self is no longer approached as a problem to be worked on, but it is not yet fully related to either. What emerges is a minimal form of contact—not structured, not named, but sustained.

Placed before *Ecstasy,* this configuration provides necessary stability. Without it, more intense affective states are either pursued or avoided. Remaining with experience without directing it allows those developments to occur without immediate disruption.

## Concluding Reflections

*Emergent Relationship* does not announce itself through insight or change. It is visible in something more restrained: the patient begins to stay with what has appeared.

There is less movement away—less explanation, less correction, less urgency to make something of the moment. What has been said is allowed to remain, even if it is incomplete. At times, this shift is accompanied by a subtle change in the quality of experience—something less defended, more continuous, not yet organized but no longer entirely withheld. It may register as a faint sense of contact, or as a loosening in how the self is held in relation to others. As Almaas (2002) describes, such moments can carry "a feeling of depth and a feeling of humanness and human connectedness," though here they appear in a more restrained form, without being developed or sustained.

This shift is easy to overlook because it lacks drama. Nothing is resolved. Nothing is clarified. But the structure of experience has altered.

The patient is no longer organized entirely around managing what arises. Nor are they yet fully able to relate to it. They remain alongside it, without withdrawing or reshaping it.

This is what prepares the ground for what follows. As experience is no longer immediately contained or redirected, it begins to intensify. What had been held at a distance starts to press forward.

What follows brings that pressure into focus.

# 19 Ecstasy

*Ecstasy* emerges in the later phases of the surrender process, when the usual organization of experience no longer holds in place. The self is not lost, but it is no longer structured by the same boundaries of time, narrative, or control.

The term retains its original meaning of *ek-stasis*—a standing outside—but here it does not refer to transcendence in a dramatic or transportive sense. Rather, it reflects a shift in how experience is registered. What had previously been contained, observed, or held in relation is no longer mediated in the same way.

Unlike satisfaction or resolution, this state is not organized around completion. It does not follow from understanding, nor does it stabilize into meaning. It appears without being produced and recedes without being retained.

In psychoanalytic terms, Bion's (1970) concept of O offers a precise framework. O cannot be known, represented, or accumulated. It is approached only under conditions in which memory, desire, and understanding are suspended. This requirement is not new, but here it reaches its limit. The structures that previously supported contact with experience are no longer sufficient to contain it.

As Wilfred Bion (1970) emphasizes, the task is not to make contact with truth as an object, but to remain in relation to what cannot be organized as knowledge. That relation comes under increased pressure. Experience is no longer shaped into something thinkable before it is felt.

What distinguishes *Ecstasy* from earlier configurations is not simply openness, but a change in structure. The individual is no longer positioned alongside experience. The distinction between observer and experience becomes less defined, and the usual organizing distance falls away.

It is in this limited sense that Heidegger's description of *ek-stasis* becomes relevant. He describes existence as always already "standing outside" itself—disclosed through time rather than contained within it (1927/1962). In *Ecstasy*, something of this structure becomes experientially apparent: the self is no longer gathered into a single, organizing position, but encountered as already beyond itself.

DOI: 10.4324/9781003795803-23

At its furthest point, this does not result in fragmentation. The self remains, but without its usual coordinating function. What occurs is not expansion in a metaphorical sense, but a temporary suspension of the structures that ordinarily maintain coherence.

This condition is easily misrecognized. Because it does not conform to familiar forms of experience, it is taken up as affect, explained through bodily states, or drawn back into interpretation. The absence of structure registers as something to be accounted for, rather than something to remain within. At other times, it is confused with regression or loss of coherence, particularly where the distinction between suspension and disorganization is not established. What differentiates this condition is not the intensity of the experience, but the absence of effort to secure it. Where this holds, the moment occurs without being extended, named, or brought into use. Where it does not, the experience is reorganized — often without recognition — into forms that restore distance and intelligibility. In this sense, *Ecstasy* does not fail when it disappears, but when it is taken up as something to be preserved or explained.

## Jerome

Jerome rarely spoke of longing. His sessions were precise, structured, controlled—as if speaking itself required careful management. He tended to stay close to what could be organized, explained, or held in place.

One afternoon, he began describing a dream. He was standing at the edge of a wide body of water. The surface was still. There was nothing to orient himself with—no path, no marker—only the sense that he could step forward without knowing where it would lead.

As he spoke, something in his delivery shifted. He did not move to interpret the dream or ask what it meant. The usual structuring of his thoughts fell away.

He paused.

His hand hovered briefly near his chest, as if registering something he had not anticipated.

"It was... peaceful," he said.

He stopped there.

A flicker crossed his face—uncertainty, then something sharper.

"I don't know what that was," he added quickly. "Probably low blood sugar or something."

He gave a short laugh and looked away.

The moment closed almost immediately. Where there had been a brief suspension of his usual organization, there was now a return to explanation—something physical, containable, dismissible.

He did not return to the dream.

## Gabriella

Gabriella's work had always moved in small increments. Where others shifted abruptly or resisted openly, her changes were less visible—registered in pauses, in tone, in what she no longer moved away from.

After a long stretch of silence in one session, she began to speak.

"I remembered something," she said. "When I was little, there was this patch of sunlight in the upstairs hallway. I used to lie in it. I'd pretend the floor was a boat, and I was floating."

She stopped.

The memory remained present in the room, not as something she was explaining, but as something she was still inside.

Her breathing had slowed. She did not look toward me to see how it would be received.

There was no movement to interpret it.

Tears gathered but did not fall. She did not wipe them away.

"I don't know why I remembered that," she said after a moment. "But it feels... good. Like it's mine."

She left it there.

The session continued, but she did not return to the memory or try to make sense of it.

## What It Asks of the Therapist

In these moments, a different demand is placed on the therapist. The task is not to deepen or clarify the patient's experience, but to avoid altering it once it has begun to unfold.

Moments of this kind are brief and easily disrupted. The pressure to respond — to name what is happening, to steady it, or to make use of it — can be strong. These impulses are recognized and held back.

With patients like Jerome, the contact is often short-lived. A moment of unmediated experience is followed quickly by reorganization—explanation, dismissal, or a return to control. In the countertransference, this can produce a pull to re-establish structure, to bring the session back into familiar analytic territory. That pull should be understood as part of the field, not acted upon.

With patients like Gabriella, the shift may be less abrupt. She may remain with the experience without developing or explaining it. Here, the countertransference may include a wish to preserve the moment, or to acknowledge it in some way. Even minimal affirmation, however, can redirect the experience into something organized and shared, rather than something she is sustaining herself.

Interpretation is not required here. Neither is encouragement. What matters is that the therapist does not move ahead of the patient by shaping what has appeared.

The task is to allow the experience to resolve on its own terms—without extending it, naming it, or drawing it into meaning.

## Justification for the Placement of this Configuration

*Ecstasy* appears in the later phases of the surrender process, following the loosening of effort in *Non-Willing* and the shift in position established in *Emergent Relationship*. By this point, the individual is no longer organizing experience through interpretation, control, or defense.

What emerges here is not something new, but something no longer mediated in the same way. Experience is not taken up, shaped, or worked on. It occurs without being organized into meaning.

Its placement reflects a change in how experience is held. The individual is no longer relating to what arises from a position alongside it, nor attempting to regulate it through understanding. The usual distance between observer and experience falls away.

There may be moments of intensity, or none at all. What distinguishes this condition is not affective tone, but the absence of interference. Experience is neither pursued nor avoided.

Its placement reflects this change. Without the prior reduction of striving and the capacity to remain with experience without organizing it, what appears is either disrupted or drawn back into interpretation.

## Concluding Reflections

*Ecstasy* does not present as a sustained state, nor does it resolve into understanding. It appears briefly, and often without warning, when the usual structures that organize experience are no longer in place.

In these moments, the individual is not working on themselves, nor relating to their experience in a deliberate way. The distinction between observer and experience becomes less defined, and what occurs is not mediated before it is felt.

The accounts of Jerome and Gabriella show two different responses to this shift. Jerome moves quickly to restore structure, re-establishing distance through explanation. Gabriella remains with the experience but does not extend or organize it. In both cases, the moment is temporary.

Ecstasy does not confirm an endpoint. It does not stabilize into a new position. It is better understood as a brief change in the organization of experience—one that cannot be maintained and does not need to be.

What appears here cannot be secured. Attempts to hold onto it risk drawing experience back into effort, organization, and control.

The experience does not remain. What may persist is not the state itself, but the fact that it occurred.

# 20 Doubt

*Doubt* emerges when the structures that previously organized experience no longer hold, and nothing has yet taken their place.

It does not present as indecision or uncertainty in the ordinary sense. Rather, it appears as a disruption in how experience is held. What had once felt stable—interpretations, convictions, even a sense of self—can no longer be relied upon in the same way.

This shift can be difficult to recognize at first. The individual may attempt to restore coherence by returning to familiar explanations or positions. When this fails, doubt begins to take on a different quality. It is no longer something to be resolved, but something that must be endured.

What is relinquished here is not only certainty, but the assumption that experience can be secured through thought, interpretation, or position. Earlier forms of knowing carried with them an implicit sense of mastery—an expectation that what was encountered could be organized, clarified, or resolved. As these structures fail, that assumption begins to loosen. The loss of omnipotence is not encountered directly, but registers through the inability to restore coherence in familiar ways. What had previously held does not return and cannot be made to return. In this sense, doubt does not introduce uncertainty so much as expose the limits of what could be known or controlled.

In this condition, the self is not reorganized so much as unsettled. What had been held together loosens, but nothing replaces it. The result is often a sense of disorientation—not collapse in every case, but a loss of certainty that cannot be immediately repaired.

This disorientation does not necessarily take the form of collapse but reflects a disturbance in the internal points of reference through which experience had been organized. Thought continues but no longer stabilizes in the same way. Interpretation may still occur but it does not hold. What had once provided a sense of coherence now fails to secure it, leaving experience without a reliable structure through which it can be taken up. In this condition, the self is not undone but is no longer able to rely on the forms that previously sustained it. What remains is a kind of exposure—without immediate disintegration, but also without the means to restore what has been lost.

DOI: 10.4324/9781003795803-24

Winnicott's (1971) observation that "It is a joy to be hidden, and disaster not to be found" becomes relevant here in a particular way. In doubt, the individual is no longer fully available to themselves. Familiar points of reference recede, and what remains cannot yet be clearly recognized or claimed.

For some, this leads to withdrawal or defensive reorganization. For others, there is a gradual shift toward remaining with the uncertainty without resolving it. The difference lies not in the presence of doubt, but in the capacity to stay with what cannot yet be understood.

## Bill

Bill measured life in things done and things still to do. He didn't talk much about feelings, only about what needed fixing or what used to be better. His sense of self had been built quietly, day by day, in jobs finished, in promises kept.

But lately, the world he had built his life around was starting to thin out. Work had dried up. His wife had stopped talking to him about anything that mattered. Friends he had known for years had moved away or got sick.

He came into a session once and sat with his hands folded, staring at the floor.

"I don't know," he said after a while. "I used to know what the hell I was supposed to be doing. There was always something. You get up, you go, you fix it, you come home."

I waited.

"Now I wake up and..." He shook his head. "There's nothing that needs me. Or if there is, I don't see it."

A pause.

"I keep thinking I'm missing something. Like I forgot what I'm supposed to be doing."

He gave a small shrug. "But I don't think I did. I think it's just... gone."

He didn't look up when he said it.

"I'm not trying to start anything new," he added after a moment. "Don't even know what that would be."

Another pause.

"Just feels like... what I had doesn't work anymore."

The room settled into it. There was no urgency in him, no reaching—only a slow recognition that something had fallen away and nothing had come to take its place.

In the countertransference, there was a thick, steady weight in the room—a sense of having to sit still in the quiet wreckage without trying to name it too soon.

## Winston

Winston had spent years hovering between collapse and survival, holding together the semblance of a life through self-deprecation, short bursts of effort, and long stretches of inertia. Therapy had begun to stabilize his rhythm: he came more regularly now, his sessions no longer punctuated by absences or last-minute cancellations. He had even resumed part-time work at a small clinic—a quieter practice than his former life demanded, but one he could sustain without imploding.

One afternoon, after describing a mundane day of seeing patients and walking home, Winston sat back and exhaled heavily.

"I don't know if it matters," he said, almost to himself. "All this effort to show up, to be a person again."

A pause.

"Some days it feels real. Other days it feels... hollow."

He didn't smile when he said it. There was no irony, no deflection—just the statement, left where it fell.

"I keep thinking it's supposed to add up to something," he said. "Like if I just keep doing it, it'll click."

He shook his head.

"But it doesn't. Not really."

Another pause.

"I'm not falling apart," he added. "I'm just... not convinced."

The moment didn't close. There was no urgency in him, but also no reassurance—only a suspended uncertainty that didn't resolve into either hope or collapse.

After a long pause, I said, "You're still here, even without it adding up."

Winston looked at me—not with skepticism, but with a tired recognition. He didn't respond. But he stayed.

## What It Asks of the Therapist

*Doubt* places the therapist in a terrain where clarity is neither available nor desirable. The task is not to resolve the patient's uncertainty, but to remain present with it—allowing disorientation and the loss of former structures to unfold without premature closure.

In Bill's case, where doubt moves toward collapse, the therapist must tolerate the patient's retreat without rushing to repair or interpret it. The work lies in bearing witness to the dismantling, trusting that remaining through the absence of structure may itself have meaning, even if nothing new has yet emerged.

With Winston, *Doubt* does not collapse but also does not resolve. The therapist is invited to recognize the patient's capacity to remain present without turning away. A simple acknowledgment—that he is still there, even without clarity or reassurance—can sustain the moment without converting it into progress. In the countertransference, the space may feel heavier, but less pressured. The pull to organize or restore meaning softens. The task is to remain there, without turning the moment into something it is not.

Across both cases, the countertransference may also evoke a strong wish to intervene—to reorient the patient, to offer meaning, to hasten resolution. This impulse must be held rather than enacted. The therapist's capacity to remain with what does not yet cohere becomes part of what holds the patient.

*Doubt* requires that the therapist relinquish the role of guide or interpreter and take up instead the role of companion: one who can stand beside the patient in a state where nothing can yet be claimed, but much is at stake.

## Justification for the Placement of this Configuration

*Doubt* follows the opening created in earlier phases such as *Emergent Relationship* and *Ecstasy*. What was experienced there—moments of openness, contact, or unguarded presence—does not hold. The patient begins to question it: whether it was real, whether it can last, whether it belongs to them at all.

This questioning does not undo surrender. It prevents the experience from hardening into something claimed or idealized. What had felt immediate becomes uncertain. The patient can no longer rely on the experience itself and must remain without knowing what it meant or whether it will return.

At this point, doubt introduces a pause. Not a retreat, but a loss of orientation. What had begun to open is no longer stable, and nothing has taken its place. The patient is left between positions—no longer held by earlier structures, but not yet able to live from what has emerged.

In this way, doubt does not signal regression. It exposes the limits of what has already been reached. What is relinquished here is not only certainty, but the expectation that experience will organize itself into something secure. What remains is the capacity to stay where nothing yet resolves.

## Concluding Reflections

*Doubt* unsettles what had begun to take shape. The beliefs and identifications that once organized experience no longer hold in the same way, but nothing has yet come to replace them. What remains is exposure—an encounter with the self that cannot be secured through certainty or meaning.

This does not move the process backward. It prevents what has been experienced from becoming fixed or claimed too quickly. The patient is left without the assurance that what felt real will return, or that it can be relied upon at all. Surrender, at this point, no longer rests on experience, but on the capacity to remain where nothing resolves.

Experiences of this kind have been described in other traditions as well. St. John of the Cross (1959) writes of a darkness in which the self is stripped of its usual supports—not as collapse, but as a condition in which familiar structures no longer hold. What remains is not clarity, but exposure.

Through the experiences of Bill and Winston, two different forms of doubt emerge: one in which the loss of structure leads toward collapse, and one in which the individual remains present, though unconvinced and without reassurance. In both, doubt does not offer resolution. It interrupts the expectation that experience will organize itself into something stable.

*Doubt* does not yield meaning, but remaining in it allows the process to continue. It depends on the individual's capacity to remain where certainty has fallen away and nothing has yet taken its place.

As this capacity develops, the work moves toward *Contemplation*, where openness can be sustained for longer periods, and then into *Foreboding*, where the anxieties bound to that openness begin to surface more fully.

# 21 Contemplation

*Contemplation* enters as attention turns inward without urgency to resolve or explain. In analytic work, it is not directed toward insight or correction but toward remaining with experience as it unfolds. Thoughts, affects, and unconscious movements are allowed to appear without immediate intervention. What has been kept out of awareness begins to show itself.

What makes this possible is not only the emergence of a new capacity, but a change in the necessity of securing experience as it appears. Earlier, what was encountered had to be organized, clarified, or resolved in order to be tolerated. As that requirement loosens, experience no longer depends on being brought into coherence to be sustained. What remains is not certainty, but the capacity to stay with what does not yet take form, without returning to the structures that once held it in place.

Psychological traditions have not always defined contemplation with the precision found in mystical writing. In Christian and Sufi texts, it is described as a movement of purification and illumination—less an achievement than a condition in which the self is encountered rather than constructed (Underhill, 1983). In the analytic setting, this appears as moments in which disowned or unformulated aspects of experience come into view before they can be organized.

Winnicott's (1971) observation that "It is a joy to be hidden, and disaster not to be found" (p. 128) again becomes relevant here. The self must be permitted a degree of obscurity if it is to emerge. In contemplation, movement toward meaning recedes. What is not yet formed is allowed to remain.

This capacity is not given. For many patients, the ability to observe without judgment—to remain with what is emerging without moving to repair, interpret, or withdraw—develops slowly. It depends on the patient's prior relation to uncertainty, absence, and psychic space. The following vignettes trace two movements: one in which the self begins to encounter itself without defense, and one in which reflection is prematurely closed.

This condition is easily disrupted. The movement toward explanation can return without being noticed, bringing experience back under forms of organization that appear reflective but function to restore coherence. What distinguishes contemplation is not the absence of thought, but the absence

DOI: 10.4324/9781003795803-25

of its necessity. Experience does not need to be clarified in order to be sustained. Where this holds, what appears is not immediately drawn back into interpretation or resolution. Where it does not, the moment closes—almost imperceptibly—and the prior relation to experience resumes.

## Gabriella

Gabriella sat with her hands folded in her lap, her gaze steady but not quite meeting mine.

"I was always the strong one," she said. "With the students. With my family." A pause. "It kept things steady."

The word remained between us.

She adjusted her hands slightly, as if resettling them. "I can see how quickly I return to that," she said. "Even here."

I didn't respond.

"It happens before I've really taken in what I'm feeling," she continued. "I move to keep things in place."

She glanced toward me briefly, then away.

"There is something else there," she said, more quietly. "But I don't give it much room."

Her posture remained composed, but her voice had shifted slightly—less certain, though no less controlled.

"It feels... unnecessary," she added after a moment. "To go further than that."

She looked toward me again, holding the gaze a second longer than before, then letting it drop.

"I think I've always believed that," she said.

She adjusted her posture, the moment settling back into something more familiar.

## Jerome

Jerome sat forward slightly in his chair, his hands folded tightly in his lap. His voice was steady, though something in it felt held in place.

"I keep thinking about who I was... and who I might be becoming," he said. "It's strange. Like I'm watching something shift, but I don't really know what it is yet."

He paused, as if waiting for it to settle into something more definite.

I didn't respond.

He nodded once, almost to himself. "There's a part of me that wants to understand it," he said. "To be able to say what's changing, or where it's going."

His gaze moved briefly toward me, then away again.

"And another part..." He stopped. "I don't want to get ahead of it."

The sentence landed differently—less certain.

He exhaled. "I just don't want to end up soft. Or lost. Or..." He caught himself. "Without some kind of structure."

The words came with more force, as if restoring something.

He shifted slightly in his chair, his posture tightening again. "There's something happening," he said. "I can't quite place it."

A pause.

"It would be easier if I could."

He glanced toward me, then straightened, his hands returning to stillness in his lap.

## What It Asks of the Therapist

*Contemplation* asks the therapist to remain present without moving the process forward. Unlike earlier configurations, the work is not to deepen or direct, but to stay with what is beginning to register without giving it form too quickly.

In Gabriella's case, where something begins to open but remains held back, the task is to leave it where it is—acknowledging it without drawing it further out or making it more explicit than she can bear. The pressure to respond, to recognize, or to meet her more fully can be felt in the room but following that pressure risks closing what has only just begun to appear.

In Jerome's case, the pull is different. As uncertainty emerges, so does the movement to define it. The therapist may feel drawn to help him articulate, to give shape to what is not yet settled. But doing so aligns with his effort to regain control. The task instead is to remain with him at the point where definition fails, without stepping in to complete it.

Across both, the countertransference often takes the form of wanting to move things along—to clarify, steady, or make use of what is appearing. Here, that movement is the intervention to resist. What is required is the capacity to remain with something not yet organized, and not to replace it with something that is.

## Justification for the Placement of this Configuration

*Contemplation* follows the disruption of *Doubt* and the opening of *Ecstasy*. Something has already been unsettled; something has already been encountered. It does not advance the process but holds it at the point where experience can be registered without being taken up too quickly.

It marks a point at which experience can remain without being organized. What has lost its certainty is not yet replaced and does not need to be. The work here is not to interpret or resolve, but to allow what has appeared to stand without being secured.

In this way, *Contemplation* extends the process of surrender by altering the individual's relation to experience itself. What develops is not only the capacity to remain, but the ability to encounter what is emerging without immediately organizing it into meaning or action.

## Concluding Reflections

Contemplation represents a maturing relation to the self—one in which the individual no longer strives for answers but remains with their own experience. Rather than resolving uncertainty, contemplation holds moments of insight, doubt, and ecstasy within an unfolding coherence. Transformation is not a singular event, but a process marked by deepening rather than arrival.

In making space for what was once obscured, the individual cultivates a more compassionate and enduring relationship to themselves, one that can bear the unfinishedness of becoming.

Through *Contemplation*, Gabriella and Jerome each come into contact with something not yet organized. Gabriella remains near it without withdrawing; Jerome moves to define it but cannot fully do so. In these moments, experience is neither resolved nor secured and does not need to be.

*Contemplation* does not ask for perfection. It asks only for presence—the quiet courage to stay near to what is forming, even when its final shape cannot yet be seen.

# 22 Foreboding

*Foreboding* is marked by a subtle but persistent sense that something remains ahead. It is not overt anxiety or acute fear, but an emerging awareness that something within the self has not yet been encountered. Within the process of surrender, it signals the presence of psychic material not yet taken up or brought into form.

Although little discussed in formal psychological literature, *Foreboding* can be understood as the self's early recognition that further surrender will require a confrontation with more complex, and potentially disorganizing, internal realities. In Bion's terms, this reflects the presence of experience that has not yet been transformed into thought but is nonetheless felt as approaching (Bion, 1962). *Foreboding*, in this light, is less a regression than a psychic preparation: an awareness that what lies ahead may unsettle, disorient, and demand a greater yielding than the self has yet endured.

When *Foreboding* arises, it is rarely met directly. More often, it stirs defensive movements—withdrawal, over-control, numbing—as the self braces against what cannot yet be faced. In some patients, foreboding leads to a turning inward; in others, to an increased effort to master. The following cases illustrate two contrasting responses to the experience of *Foreboding*: one muted, one driven, each shaped by the particular vulnerabilities of the inner world.

## Bill

Bill arrived early for his session, settling into the chair with a stiffness that seemed to press down on him. When I asked how he had been, he shrugged.

"Fine. Same old," he said.

"What's been taking up your time?"

"Nothing much." He paused. "Fixed a cabinet door. It kept swinging open."

"What was wrong with it?"

"Loose hinge." He looked down at his hands. "Tightened it. For now."

A brief silence.

DOI: 10.4324/9781003795803-26

"Back steps are still off," he added. "There's a board that shifts when you step on it."

"You notice it when you walk over it?"

"Yeah." He nodded. "Not enough to fix. Just... there." He gave a small shrug. "You forget about it, then it catches you."

He glanced up briefly, then away again.

"Watched something last night," he continued. "Didn't really follow it."

"What was it?"

"Don't know. Some show." A pause. "Left it on."

Bill shifted slightly in his chair. "Something's off," he said. "I don't know where."

He let out a short breath. "It's stupid."

"Saying that?"

He shook his head. "Just... saying that." A faint smile, quick and gone. "Probably just tired."

"Different?"

Bill didn't answer right away. He rubbed his thumb along the edge of his hand.

"I don't know," he said finally. "I can't point to anything."

He sat with that for a moment, then shifted again.

"Anyway," he added, a little more briskly, "I should probably fix that board before someone trips."

He sat there a moment, then said something about the weather.

## Jerome

Jerome entered the session with a restless energy, speaking almost before he sat down.

"I sent that report before anyone else could get theirs in," he said. "And I got in early every day this week—like, earlier than I needed to. Just to get ahead of things."

He adjusted his sleeve, then continued.

"And I went back through the deadlines again last night. Just to make sure nothing shifted."

"What would happen if something did?" I asked.

He gave a quick, dismissive exhale. "It won't. That's the point."

A brief pause.

"I just don't want to miss anything important," he added, half-laughing. "If I stay ahead of it, I'm good."

"What is the 'it'?"

Jerome's eyes flicked toward me, then away. His foot began tapping against the floor.

"I mean—anything," he said. "Stuff changes. People drop things. You've got to be ready."

"Ready for what?"

His jaw tightened slightly. "Just... not to get caught off guard."

I let that sit.

His tapping slowed, then picked up again.

"Because once you are," he added, more quietly, "you're already behind."

The room shifted. Not dramatically—but enough.

Jerome leaned forward, elbows on his knees, as if trying to regain ground.

"It's just how things work," he said. "You either stay ahead or you're reacting. And reacting's too late."

## What It Asks of the Therapist

*Foreboding* tests the therapist's ability to remain with something that has not yet taken shape. It does not present as clear anxiety or identifiable conflict. In Bill, it appears as a sense that something is off, without being locatable. In Jerome, it takes the form of urgency—an effort to stay ahead of something he cannot name.

In both, the pressure is to move too quickly: to clarify, to organize, to make sense of what is only beginning to register.

The task is to resist that movement.

This requires what Bion (1962) described as the capacity to work without memory or desire—to stay with the patient's experience without reaching for explanation or resolution. The therapist must be able to register the shift in the room without converting it into meaning too soon.

At this point, interpretation can function as a defense. Naming what is happening risks closing down the very process that is trying to emerge. What is needed instead is a sustained tolerance for what feels unfinished, indirect, or misplaced.

*Foreboding* often stirs something similar in the therapist: a pull to steady the moment, to make it coherent. The work is to recognize that pull without acting on it—to remain in contact with the patient without organizing the experience on their behalf.

## Justification for the Placement of this Configuration

*Foreboding* follows *Contemplation* as the work begins to shift from observing experience to encountering what has not yet been taken in. Reflection no longer holds the same distance. Something unsettled starts to press forward.

It does not arrive as clear anxiety or defined conflict. Instead, there is a sense that something remains unresolved—felt but not located, approaching but not yet known. This signals that earlier understanding has not yet reached the deeper layers now coming into range.

For this reason, *Foreboding* interrupts any premature sense of completion. It introduces a form of tension that cannot be resolved through reflection alone. What has been seen can no longer be held at a distance.

Although *Foreboding* may return throughout the process, it may reappear in similar or altered form, depending on what has and has not yet been taken in. Each re-emergence reflects a further reworking of what has not yet been fully taken in.

Bion's (1971/2014) conception of the grid offers a way of understanding this movement: meaning is not fixed but continually reclassified as new emotional realities come into contact with the mind. What has been thought must be thought again, differently, as deeper layers come into view.

By allowing this unease to remain, rather than moving to settle it, the individual becomes able to stay with what is not yet formed. In this way, *Foreboding* marks the point at which reflection no longer organizes experience, and something more demanding begins to emerge.

## Concluding Reflections

*Foreboding* does not resolve into understanding. It introduces a shift in the work—one that cannot be managed through reflection, preparation, or control.

In Bill, this appeared as something off, without location. In Jerome, as the need to stay ahead of something that could not be named. In both, the experience remained just out of reach, yet increasingly difficult to ignore.

What emerges at this point is not clarity, but pressure. Something begins to register that has not yet taken form and cannot be organized in the ways that have previously held.

Attempts to steady the experience—through explanation, withdrawal, or control—do not resolve it. They only mark the limits of what can be managed.

*Foreboding* does not tell the patient what is coming. It establishes that something is.

And that it will require more than what has brought them this far.

# Part IV

# Releasement Level C

## Living Coherence: The Circulatory and Endocrine Functions of Psychic Life

After disruption settles, a different form of coherence may be observed. *Releasement Level C* encompasses configurations in which the psyche begins to inhabit changes that have come into view. What once appeared as insight or rupture comes to be lived as a way of moving through the world. The individual is no longer metabolizing experience in order to change—it is the change that moves within them.

The configurations in this level—*Shift, Gratitude, Love, Wisdom, Revealing, Unconcealment, Dynamic Flow,* and *Repetition*—are not endpoints. They are lived rhythms. Rather than signifying completion, they reflect a return to life from within a differently organized internal world. A patient may still struggle, still revisit earlier fears or defenses, but these occur within a context that can hold, metabolize, and re-form experience with greater fluidity.

Anatomically, this level corresponds to the body's circulatory and endocrine systems—those associated with sustaining internal rhythm, continuity, and hormonal regulation. These configurations do not proceed in a straight line; they recur and reconfigure, revealing new dimensions each time. They are not achievements but patterns of return—indications that the psyche is no longer only surviving or relinquishing control but participating in its own ongoing organization.

Neurobiologically, this level can be understood as involving a more coordinated relationship among affective, cognitive, and autonomic systems. In contexts where a degree of internal coherence is present, there may be more stable regulation across processes associated with the hypothalamic-pituitary-adrenal (HPA) axis and vagal tone, alongside increased flexibility in responding to stress and affective demand. The individual may be able to move between states without the same degree of disorganization—shifting between feeling and reflection, intimacy and autonomy, rupture and repair. This rhythm is not fixed or complete, but remains dynamic, subject to disruption, and open to further reorganization.

DOI: 10.4324/9781003795803-27

# 23 Shift

*Shift* refers to a change that does not occur through the processes described in Releasement Level B. It is not built through reflection or gradual insight, but arrives more abruptly—often experienced as a release within the body that alters how previously entrenched issues are held. What had been approached through effort or understanding begins to reorganize without the same degree of conscious management.

This movement differs from what precedes in a decisive way. Earlier, the work involved a reduction of effort—less organization, less anticipation, less need to secure what was encountered. Here, experience reorganizes without being acted upon. What had been loosened does not remain open but alters its configuration without deliberate intervention. The individual does not arrive at this change through reflection or decision. It takes place within the experience itself and is recognized only after it has begun. In this sense, *Shift* does not extend the work of relinquishment. It marks the point at which something reorganizes in its absence.

From a psychoanalytic perspective, this can be understood as a reallocation of psychic energy: what had been bound in defense or held in tension begins to loosen, allowing new configurations of experience to emerge. The change is not primarily cognitive. It is registered in how the individual feels, responds, and inhabits their internal world.

Following a *Shift*, the individual may find that new forms of experience become possible—gratitude, love, or wisdom—not as efforts to be cultivated, but as states that begin to arise on their own. In this sense, *Shift* does not complete the process. It alters the conditions under which further movement becomes possible.

## Jerome

Jerome was in the middle of describing a week that had gone well—deadlines met early, a case he felt confident about, a meeting he had anticipated and handled cleanly.

"I like knowing where things are headed," he said. "If I stay ahead of it, there's no scrambling."

DOI: 10.4324/9781003795803-28

He paused.

"It's always been like that," he added.

"Always?" I asked.

He nodded. "Yeah." He paused again. When he continued, his tone had changed. "Even now. I was at my mom's last weekend—same thing. I got there early, helped her get things set up before anyone else showed up." A small shrug. "It just makes things easier."

He continued, still measured. "I remember doing that when I was younger too. Making sure things were... handled." He stopped.

His hand moved to his chest, almost absently. He looked down, then closed his eyes for a moment.

"What's happening?" I asked.

He shook his head slightly. "I don't know." A pause. "It's... strange."

He stayed there, quieter now. His breathing slowed.

"It feels like something just... dropped," he said. "Or let go."

I didn't respond.

He opened his eyes but didn't look at me right away. His shoulders, usually held in a kind of contained readiness, had softened.

"I used to think if I didn't stay on top of everything, something would fall apart," he said. "Not in a dramatic way. Just... things would slip."

He frowned slightly.

"I don't feel that right now."

Another pause.

"It's not the situation," he said. "It's how I am in it." He looked up, almost checking. "I'm not... managing it."

I stayed with him.

He let out a short breath. "That's new."

After a moment, he glanced over at me. "You're not going to tell me what that means?"

There was a familiar pull in it—toward clarity, toward getting ahead of the experience.

"I don't think this moment needs that yet," I said.

He held my gaze, then nodded once.

"Yeah," he said. "It doesn't."

He leaned back slightly, not withdrawing—just less braced.

"For once," he added, "I don't feel like I have to stay ahead of it."

We sat there for a bit longer without speaking.

The change did not come through effort or understanding. It registered first as a release in the body, and only afterward in how he related to what had previously required control. What shifted was not the memory itself, but the necessity to stay ahead of it.

## Gabriella

Gabriella spoke about her granddaughter, describing the way the child would come to her without hesitation.

"She just climbs right into my lap," she said, a small smile forming. "Like she knows I'll hold her."

She paused.

Her hand moved toward her abdomen, almost protectively.

"She doesn't think about it," she added. "She just… comes."

Her voice caught slightly. She looked down.

"I never did that," she said after a moment. "Not with my mother." A small shake of her head. "I don't think I ever let anyone do that with me."

I waited.

She seemed to notice something in her own body—her arms, folded tightly across her chest. Slowly, she let them fall open into her lap.

"I always thought it was enough to be kind," she said. "To not need too much." A pause. "That that was… better."

She looked up briefly, then away again.

"But I think I've been hiding," she said, more quietly. "Behind that."

"And now?" I asked.

She hesitated, as if the next words required permission.

"I think…" She stopped, then tried again. "I think I'd like to be held too."

Her eyes filled, but she did not look away.

I didn't respond.

She remained there, not retracting, not softening the statement.

After a moment, she exhaled.

"That feels strange to say," she said. "But not wrong."

We sat with it.

The change did not arrive as insight, but as a loosening of a long-held relational position. What had been organized around not needing began to give way to the possibility of receiving. The shift was subtle, but it altered the direction of her speech—from offering to allowing herself to want.

## What It Asks of the Therapist

*Shift* places a particular demand on the therapist—the capacity not to move in too quickly. These moments are not declared. They register first in small changes—in how the patient speaks, where they stop, what they no longer try to manage.

The task is not to interpret, and not to stabilize what is happening. It is to remain with it.

Bion's concept of reverie (1962) is useful here, not as a technique but as a discipline. The therapist receives the moment without organizing it—holding their own impulse to name, clarify, or make use of it.

In both Gabriella's and Jerome's sessions, the movement occurred when the therapist did not take over the experience. With Jerome, this meant not answering the pull toward explanation. With Gabriella, it meant not softening or redirecting the emergence of want. In each case, the shift held because it was not immediately shaped.

These moments are easily lost. If they are interpreted too quickly, they become insight. If they are affirmed too directly, they risk becoming performance. The therapist's restraint allows the experience to register before it is understood.

What follows is not necessarily language, but a change in how the patient occupies their experience. From there, other movements may become possible—not through effort, but because something has already reorganized.

## Justification for the Placement of this Configuration

*Shift* follows *Doubt, Contemplation,* and *Foreboding*—configurations in which the usual ways of organizing experience loosen. Certainty is disrupted, experience is held without immediate explanation, and what emerges can no longer be fully managed or anticipated.

*Shift* does not occur through effort. It appears when that work has already taken place—often at a point where nothing new is being pursued.

What distinguishes this from the preceding movements is not simply that effort has diminished, but that processes of loosening and suspension no longer define the experience. In *Doubt* and *Contemplation,* the individual remains in relation to what cannot be organized, sustaining a condition in which prior structures no longer hold. That condition gives way to a reorganization that does not depend on continued openness or endurance. What had been unsettled does not remain in suspension but alters its form without being worked on. *Shift* is not a continuation of those configurations, but a change in how experience moves once the necessity of holding or maintaining it has fallen away.

What matters here is not insight, but a release of the need to remain ahead of the experience. Something that had been held in place—through control, restraint, or quiet compliance—gives way.

Christopher Bollas' (1987) concept of the unthought known is useful here. What emerges in a shift is not necessarily something newly discovered, but something that had not yet been lived in this way. It becomes real not through articulation, but through a change in how it is held.

*Shift* is a change in position. The individual is no longer relating to experience as something to manage or understand, but as something they can remain within. From here, later developments—*Gratitude, Love, Wisdom*—do not need to be pursued. They arise from what has already begun.

## Concluding Reflections

*Shift* becomes evident in how the patient no longer needs to manage what is unfolding. What had required holding or anticipation begins to give way.

What changes is not what the patient knows, but how they are situated in relation to it. The pressure to organize, anticipate, or contain gives way, and something previously held at a distance becomes livable.

For Jerome, this appears as a release from staying ahead—no longer needing to manage what is unfolding. For Gabriella, it takes the form of allowing want to emerge without immediately softening or withdrawing it. In each case, the movement is small but decisive: something is no longer being held in the same way.

This does not resolve the process. It alters it.

What follows may deepen into gratitude, love, or wisdom—but it may also lead into further exposure, repetition, or disorientation. *Shift* does not determine the direction. It makes further movement possible.

Something has changed in how experience can be borne. And once that change has occurred, it cannot be entirely undone.

# 24 Gratitude

*Gratitude* represents an inwardly transformative condition in the surrender process—one that extends beyond appreciation into the realm of psychic integration. It arises not simply from feeling thankful, but from the internal recognition of goodness—within oneself, in the other, and in the relational field that made the surrender process possible. Typically emerging after a significant shift, gratitude marks a deepening of the self's capacity to hold complexity: to acknowledge what was endured, to metabolize what was given, and to begin to receive without defense.

While the words gratitude and thankfulness are often used interchangeably, they reflect different levels of experience. Thankfulness may express appreciation for favorable conditions—health, safety, stability, even therapeutic progress. Gratitude, by contrast, reflects a relational and intrapsychic shift: the capacity to take in goodness, often after ambivalence has been tolerated or repair has been possible. Within the surrender process, gratitude is not the endpoint but a form of opening—a recognition of having been changed by contact with the self and with another.

In psychoanalytic terms, gratitude is often considered a reparative affect—a movement toward mending the inner world after conflict, ambivalence, or mourning. Melanie Klein (1957) understood gratitude as a developmental milestone: the infant's capacity to perceive the nurturing figure as good, not idealized, and to bear the accompanying feelings of dependence, love, and guilt. This capacity emerges alongside, and in tension with, envy—the impulse to diminish or control what is experienced as good—requiring the ability to take in goodness without attacking its source. It becomes the basis for future intimacy, trust, and self-worth. In the therapeutic setting, gratitude may signal a shift in how the patient relates to the therapist—not as an idealized figure, but as one who can be relied upon and emotionally encountered across time (Winnicott, 1965).

Gratitude, in this light, is not a static sentiment but a dynamic, internal act of acknowledgment: of what has been endured, what has been survived, and what is now possible. It reflects what Ogden (2005) characterizes as "a coming-into-being of experience"—a surfacing of emotional life once held at a distance. In this way, gratitude allows the individual to reclaim aspects

DOI: 10.4324/9781003795803-29

of the self once split off or devalued. It becomes not the end of surrender, but the beginning of a more fully inhabited self—one capable of openness, tenderness, and ongoing internal movement.

## Winston

Winston rarely spoke about money unless it was to downplay its meaning. A physician from an old Boston family, he lived in a dilapidated house that he sometimes shared with near-strangers. He dressed plainly, kept few possessions, and prided himself on needing little.

"I'm low-maintenance," he said once, with a faint smile. "Like a lawn."

In one session, he mentioned a recent disbursement from the family trust.

"It's enough to buy a mansion and never work again," he said. "But I'm grateful I've still got the house." A small shrug. "Keeps me grounded."

He paused, then added, almost as an afterthought, "Too much space isn't good for anyone."

I didn't respond.

He glanced toward the bookshelf.

"And I guess coming here helps with that too," he said. "Keeps the floor from falling out."

His tone was light, almost offhand. He didn't look at me as he spoke.

A few moments passed.

"You ever notice that?" he added. "People get more, and then they just… float off."

I said nothing.

He shifted slightly in his chair, then continued.

"Someone at work just bought a place on the lake," he said. "Huge. Ugly as hell." A brief pause. "I'm sure she's grateful. Somewhere to show off."

He leaned back, his gaze drifting toward the window.

Silence gathered.

After a moment, he let out a short breath, almost a laugh.

"Grateful," he said again, more quietly this time. "That's the word, right?"

I remained where I was.

He didn't look at me.

The word grateful remained in the room, untethered.

What Winston called gratitude remained organized around what could be held in place. It acknowledged what he had but did not draw him into relation with it. Nothing in his expression required him to yield or to be changed by the moment. If anything, the language of gratitude helped stabilize a position he could maintain. In this way, his thankfulness remained intact. Gratitude, as it unfolds in the surrender process, begins where one can no longer remain untouched by what is received.

## Gabriella

After a long break from in-person sessions during the COVID lockdowns, Gabriella returned to the office with a bright, almost effervescent energy. She stepped inside smiling, her eyes lively behind her mask.

"It showed up in late March," she said, settling into the chair. "Tiny, noisy, completely unbothered by me." A small laugh. "I started talking to it while I made coffee. Not that I didn't have people to talk to—I've been talking to you, obviously. But it was different. It felt nice to have something right there."

She glanced around the room.

"I actually missed this place," she added. Then, more quickly, "Missed you, too, I think."

She continued—about the bird, about the odd comfort of having something consistent just outside her window, about the relief of being back in a room with another person. As she spoke, she slipped off her coat and folded it carefully over the arm of the couch, smoothing it once, then again.

"It's strange," she said, still moving. "I thought I was fine. I mean—I was fine."

I didn't respond.

Her hands slowed. She looked down at her sleeve, smoothing it once more, but without urgency.

"It's not just the space," she said after a moment. "I felt something when I came in." A pause. "Like my body knew where it was before my mind caught up."

She looked toward me, then away again.

"I've been fine—really," she said, more softly now. "But sitting here…" She stopped, searching briefly. "It's like something lets go."

I remained where I was.

Her eyes filled slightly. She turned her head toward the window, blinking once, as if to steady herself.

"I didn't know I'd missed being met."

She didn't continue.

The room held.

After a while, she spoke again, but more slowly now.

"I don't have to explain as much," she said. "Or… get it right."

I said nothing.

She nodded faintly, as if confirming something to herself.

When the session ended, she didn't move immediately. She stood, then paused, her hand resting lightly on the back of the chair.

"I'll see you next week," she said, without urgency.

What emerged in Gabriella was not an expression of gratitude, but a shift in her capacity to receive. The contact did not require amplification or reassurance. It was registered and allowed. In contrast to earlier moments, she did not move to secure the connection or define it. She remained within it. Gratitude, here, was not spoken—it took form in her ability to stay, to be met, and to be affected without retreat.

## What It Asks of the Therapist

For the therapist, gratitude calls for an attuned restraint—an ability to recognize when something meaningful is emerging without interrupting its formation. *Gratitude*, when it arises in therapy, is rarely declared outright. It often appears obliquely: in a softened tone, a spontaneous tear, the absence of defensiveness where it once lived. It can shimmer at the edge of language, requiring the therapist to register it before it is spoken.

This condition asks the therapist to tolerate a particular form of emotional tenderness. When gratitude surfaces, it often arrives alongside grief, ambivalence, and the pain of having needed something one did not always have. When gratitude is received too eagerly, it flattens; interpreted too quickly, it retreats. The task is to hold it—allowing the patient to remain in contact with the experience long enough for it to become their own. As Klein observed, "We frequently encounter expressions of gratitude which turn out to be prompted mainly by feelings of guilt," noting that even in its most genuine forms, gratitude is tangled with the early vicissitudes of need, deprivation, and the desire to preserve the object (Klein, 1957/1975, p. 189).

Gabriella's shift into gratitude unfolded gradually. Her initial brightness masked something more fragile beneath—something she only allowed herself to feel when the room was familiar again. The therapist said little, sensing that what mattered was not the meaning of her words but the fact that she could stay in the experience without fleeing. Her gratitude was not directed at the therapist but moved through her—an emotional contact that required presence, not explanation.

By contrast, Winston's use of thankfulness operated defensively. His words gestured toward appreciation, but what they avoided was more telling: the threat of being moved. Winston's thankfulness, while not insincere, remained structurally removed from emotional contact. It was directed toward what could be owned, contained, or narrated—never toward what might involve dependency or risk. His comment about therapy floated without tether; the house remained his anchor. If there was envy, it had already been relocated—lodged in the colleague, displaced from view.

This presence—of the therapist as both witness and participant—has transformative implications. Klein described gratitude as arising only when the internalization of the good object has not been too compromised by envy: "Gratitude is rooted in the emotions and attitudes that arise in the earliest stage of infancy," she wrote, and "the individual becomes able to share its gifts with others" (Klein, 1957/1975, p. 187–188). The therapist's capacity to receive—not claim—what the patient offers is what allows gratitude to unfold without being spoiled.

Gratitude cannot be summoned by therapeutic effort, only met when it arrives. Its presence is bodily, uncertain, and sometimes brief. The realization of gratitude will be visceral—tangled with grief, receptivity, and a tender destabilization. What it asks of the therapist is not intervention, but containment: a willingness to be present without possessing, to let the patient feel the fullness of being received without being overwhelmed by it.

## Justification for the Placement of this Configuration

*Gratitude* arises within the larger movement of surrender, often following configurations such as *Doubt, Foreboding, Contemplation,* or *Shift*. It is not a reward or endpoint, but a condition in which the individual begins to feel what has been received—internally, relationally, or psychically. Rather than being achieved, it emerges as a consequence of releasing certain defenses and encountering something real.

At this point in the surrender process, the individual has begun to relinquish the illusion of control and to metabolize the impact of having been accompanied. Gratitude may appear not as a grand declaration, but as a trace affect—a softening, a slowing down, a fleeting receptivity. It signals a growing capacity to tolerate having needed and been met, however incompletely.

Melanie Klein's framing of gratitude as a reparative position is useful here, particularly in contrast to envy, which seeks to disavow the good in the other in order to preserve self-sufficiency. Gratitude, by contrast, requires a loosening of omnipotence and an openness to being touched by something beyond the self. It marks a change from defensive posture to relational presence (Klein, 1957/1975, pp. 187–188).

Ghent (1990) draws a crucial distinction between masochistic submission and genuine surrender. Where submission seeks to control the other through unconscious compliance, surrender opens the individual to a deeper inner freedom. In this light, gratitude is not about pleasing or yielding—it's what arises when the self remains intact even as it is moved. It is not a loss of agency, but a deepening of presence. And it is in this delicate balance—being affected without collapsing—that gratitude reveals itself not just as emotion, but as a reconfiguration of the self.

In the broader surrender process, gratitude anchors what has begun to change. It allows the self to begin living in relation to what has been received, rather than defending against it. It is not the end of surrender, but one of its most intimate movements.

## Concluding Reflections

*Gratitude* signals not closure but integration. It does not arrive with clarity or confidence, but with a subtle inner change—when the self, having relinquished certain defenses, begins to register what has been received. It is not the feeling of being 'lucky', nor a polite thankfulness, but something slower, more destabilizing: the recognition that one has been accompanied, and that this accompaniment has altered how experience is taken in.

Gratitude reflects a capacity to internalize goodness without evacuating ambivalence. It does not present as a stable state. It becomes available unevenly, often indirectly, and only to the extent that what has been received can be borne without immediate retreat or reorganization. It is registered less in what is declared than in what is no longer warded off.

Across patients, this capacity varies in form and degree. Gabriella comes closer to it but does not settle there. When it emerges, it is accompanied by hesitation—by the risk that allowing it will place something of herself in the other's hands. She remains, at times, where she might previously have withdrawn, but the contact is not secured. What has been received is only partially tolerated and easily complicated by the pull to reduce its impact.

Winston, by contrast, can articulate gratitude more readily, but without corresponding internal contact. He speaks it—sometimes quickly, sometimes insistently—but the expression does not hold. It moves outward, carrying the form of gratitude while preserving distance from its implications. What would need to be taken in remains unassimilated, and the experience does not consolidate.

These differences do not define fixed positions. The capacity for gratitude shifts, advances, recedes. It is contingent on what can be taken in without destabilizing the structures that have organized the self. To register that something has been received is also to encounter the fact of having depended—and of not having secured that experience alone.

Gratitude is not granted, and it cannot be prescribed. It must be discovered—often to the patient's own surprise—and tolerated long enough to be felt. Its arrival can be disarming. It may be accompanied by grief, by exposure, by a tension between taking in and pushing away.

When it appears, the task is not to name it. The analyst does not confirm it, organize it, or translate it into understanding too quickly. The work is to remain with it as it is—without foreclosing it, without converting it into something more coherent than the patient can sustain. What matters is that it is not diverted. That it is allowed to register, however partially, and to remain in the room long enough to begin to take hold.

# 25 Love

*Love*, within this phase of the surrender process, does not emerge through intention. It appears indirectly, as something that becomes possible once certain forms of holding on have been relinquished. What shifts is not only the relation to the other, but the terms under which the self is encountered—less defended against, less organized through opposition. The experience is often unfamiliar in its texture. It does not carry the urgency of need or the certainty of idealization. It holds, instead, a form of contact that can be sustained without immediate correction.

In the clinical setting, *Love* does not resemble its colloquial or romantic forms. It is not driven by fusion, nor by the need to secure the other. It takes shape as a capacity to remain in contact—both with oneself and with the other—without immediate distortion. This becomes possible only after some degree of surrender to internal reality has occurred, where aspects of the self that were previously disavowed or managed can be approached without the same level of interference.

Freud's observation that the cure is effected by love can be understood here without amplification. What comes into view is not simply a redirection of feeling, but a shift in how experience is taken in. As defensive structures loosen, something of the self becomes more accessible—not as an achievement, but as something no longer held at a distance. The change is subtle but consequential: the self can be encountered without the same pressure to revise, improve, or withdraw from what is found.

This capacity does not arise in isolation. It depends on earlier shifts that make such contact tolerable. Where what is received is met with suspicion or diminished upon entry, it cannot be retained. As this balance alters, even slightly, the possibility emerges that what comes from outside the self can be taken in without immediate undoing. Under these conditions, what has been received may begin to be held, and, over time, valued. The capacity for gratitude and the capacity for love remain closely linked—not as a sequence, but as mutually dependent conditions.

*Love*, then, is not a stable acquisition. It does not resolve conflict or secure the self against loss. It remains contingent, subject to fluctuation, and closely tied to what can be tolerated internally. At times it appears as a form

DOI: 10.4324/9781003795803-30

of recognition—of oneself, of the other—that does not require immediate stabilization. At other times it recedes, displaced by more familiar organizations of defense.

Its significance lies less in its intensity than in its conditions. Where it appears, even briefly, something has shifted in what can be borne. The self is no longer required to organize against its own experience to the same extent. What becomes possible is a form of contact that does not depend on control and does not collapse under the presence of need.

## Winston

Winston arrived late, as he often did, not apologizing. His shirt was wrinkled, collar slightly turned. He dropped into the chair with a soft exhale, running a hand through his hair as if to settle himself, then stopping halfway through the motion.

"Sorry," he said, though without emphasis. "Elevator was… doing something strange."

He smiled faintly, then let it go. The room quieted more quickly than usual.

"I had a dream," he said.

He didn't elaborate right away. His gaze moved toward the window, then back again.

"I was a kid. In a hospital waiting room. My mom was there—she was digging through her bag, looking for change." He paused. "She kept checking, like maybe she'd missed it the first time."

His fingers traced the seam of the chair.

"I remember thinking I should help her. Like, I knew I should." A slight shrug. "But I didn't move. I just… watched her."

Silence gathered, but he didn't rush to fill it.

"It felt familiar," he added, more quietly. "That part."

Another pause.

"It was the first time I didn't hate him."

I didn't respond immediately.

"Who?" I asked.

"Myself."

He shifted in his seat, then stilled again. No smile this time.

"I mean—" He stopped. "Usually I would. Or I'd make it into something. Like—what kind of person just sits there?" A brief glance upward. "But this time it was just… that's what happened."

I stayed with him, not moving to clarify.

Winston let out a small breath.

"I'm not saying I feel good about it," he said. "It's not like that." Another pause. "But I didn't feel like I had to go after him for it either."

He rubbed his face briefly. "It's weird. I'm probably making it sound like something it's not."

His voice flattened slightly on the last phrase, as if pulling back from what had just come closer.

"I didn't feel like disappearing," he said, quickly. Then, almost immediately: "I mean—I probably would've. Just not right then."

After a moment, I said, "You didn't move away."

Winston gave a short laugh—more reflex than amusement.

"Yeah. I guess." He leaned back, then forward again, elbows on his knees. "We'll see how long that lasts."

He checked the clock, though there was still time left. His foot tapped once against the floor, then stopped.

The session slowed again. He didn't pick up a new thread.

After a while, he stood, a bit abruptly. "Alright," he said, as if concluding something.

At the door, he paused—not turning back but not leaving immediately either. Then he shook his head lightly, as if dismissing something, and stepped out.

A shift occurs in Winston's relation to himself, but it does not consolidate. The reduction in hostility is brief and unstable, quickly qualified and partially withdrawn. Contact is made but not sustained. The capacity to remain with his experience without attack appears momentarily, then recedes. No symbolic reorganization follows. What is possible here is limited to a transient softening, without integration.

## Jerome

Jerome entered and closed the door more carefully than usual. He remained standing for a moment, as if deciding where to begin, then sat and adjusted his sleeve, smoothing it twice before letting his hand fall.

He didn't speak.

I waited.

After a while, he looked up.

"I've been thinking about you."

He said it plainly, then shifted in his chair.

"In a contained way," he said quickly. "I want to be precise about that."

"Not in a way that would require… concern," he added. A brief, controlled smile. "I'm aware of how that sounds."

He glanced toward the bookshelf, then back again.

"It started after last week. When I told you about the fight with my brother." A pause. "You didn't do what people usually do."

I didn't respond.

"You didn't try to fix it. Or turn it into something useful." His jaw tightened slightly. "You just said, 'That must've felt unbearable.'"

He repeated the word more quietly.

"Unbearable."

His fingers pressed lightly into his palm, as if testing it.

"I kept hearing it afterward." He exhaled through his nose. "Not like remembering. More like it... stayed active."

A small pause.

"I didn't like that." A faint shake of his head. "It felt... uncontained."

He shifted, straightening his posture.

"I tried to think it through. Figure out what it was doing there." A brief glance toward me. "Whether it was something I'd imposed. Or..." He stopped. "Something else."

Silence held.

"And then I noticed I wasn't pushing it out the way I normally would." He gave a short exhale. "Which is not typical."

I stayed with him.

"It wasn't intrusive," he said after a moment. "That's what's strange." A slight narrowing of his eyes. "It didn't feel like something I had to remove."

He leaned back, then forward again.

"I'm trying to be careful about how I say this," he added. "Because I don't want to overstate it."

Another pause.

"But there's something about... how you were with me in that moment." He stopped, recalibrating. "It didn't require anything from me. And it didn't... diminish me either."

He looked down, then back up.

"I'm not used to that."

Silence.

"I don't have a clean term for it," he said. "Which I'm not entirely comfortable with."

I said, "You're not settling it."

He let out a small breath.

"For now," he said. "I'm not committing to that."

A faint shift at the corner of his mouth—something close to humor but not fully claimed.

"I'm not convinced that's sustainable."

He adjusted his sleeve again, though it no longer needed it.

"But I didn't move it out," he added. "That's... new."

He straightened his cuff again, more precisely this time.

The room held there.

After a while, he stood, more slowly than usual. At the door, he paused briefly, as if something might still be said, then left.

Jerome approaches an experience he cannot fully define. His movement toward contact is accompanied by efforts to delimit and assess it. The reliance on mastery remains active but is no longer immediate. The experience is permitted to persist without full organization, though not yet held without qualification. What appears is a partial suspension of control, without relinquishment of it.

### What It Asks of the Therapist

To accompany a patient into the territory of *Love*, the therapist is required to tolerate a form of involvement that does not resolve into clarity. The work no longer centers on interpreting defenses or organizing meaning, but on remaining present as something less structured begins to emerge. The therapist may find themselves affected in ways that do not immediately lend themselves to use—something registers, but cannot yet be made thinkable or acted upon. What appears is not something to deepen or secure, but something to remain alongside without interference.

With Winston, the therapist's experience may be shaped as much by absence as by presence. When he says, "I didn't hate him," there can be a sense of something shifting—briefly—but without continuity. It may register as a softening, or a reduction in his usual self-attack, but it does not hold. As he qualifies the moment, moves away from it, or undercuts it, the therapist may notice how quickly the experience disperses.

When the therapist asks, "Who?", the response—"Myself"—may not open into relation. The moment remains contained within Winston. The therapist might register a faint pull toward him, alongside the recognition that the contact does not extend outward. There is no clear inclusion of the therapist in that shift. The experience appears but does not develop.

In such moments, the therapist may feel an impulse to mark or steady what has emerged—to give it form, or to hold it in place. The work is to refrain from doing so. What Winston can sustain is limited, and the therapist's task is to allow the moment to remain transient—present, then gone—without organizing it into something more stable than it is.

With Jerome, the therapist may encounter a different configuration. Contact does not recede; it is approached and then immediately subjected to control. When Jerome speaks of thinking about the therapist, and then qualifies it, the therapist may register being brought into the patient's experience, but only provisionally. The recognition is present, though not relinquished to.

There may be a sense of being held in mind—of being carried between sessions—alongside an awareness of the pressure to define and delimit that experience. When Jerome describes the persistence of the therapist's words, the therapist might register the impact of that presence, while also noticing how quickly it becomes subject to evaluation, containment, or reorganization.

In these moments, the therapist may feel pulled toward clarification—to refine what is being said, to participate in shaping it, or to meet Jerome at the level of precision he is establishing. The work is to resist that pull. To remain just outside the organizing movement, acknowledging what is present without assisting in its consolidation.

The therapist's experience here may be less one of intensity than of constraint. Something is taking place that cannot yet be fully received. It is approached, tested, and partially allowed, but not stabilized. The therapist must tolerate being included without becoming fixed, and must remain present without contributing to the structuring of the experience.

Across both cases, the therapist is asked to hold proximity without assuming its meaning. What appears as contact may dissolve, fragment, or become subject to control. The therapist cannot rely on recognition as evidence of integration, and must instead attend to what is sustained, what is withdrawn, and what remains only briefly accessible. These moments do not represent the full capacity for *Love*, but points along its emergence—where contact becomes possible under different constraints. What appears in one patient may dissolve, while in another it is held only through qualification or control.

In these moments, the therapist does not name *Love*, does not confirm it, and does not organize it. The task is more limited: to remain present as the patient encounters something they cannot yet fully use. Whether it appears as a fleeting reduction in hostility or a carefully managed recognition of the other, the therapist holds position—without amplifying, without withdrawing, and without imposing form where none can yet be maintained.

## Justification for the Placement of this Configuration

*Love* can arise under the conditions established in *Gratitude* and *Shift* but does not simply extend them. Where *Gratitude* allows for the recognition of something received, *Love* involves a different relation to that recognition—one in which it can be held without immediate qualification, reversal, or loss. It is not a movement from absence to presence, but a change in how what has been taken in is related to over time.

*Gratitude* establishes the possibility of internalizing something experienced as good without evacuating ambivalence. *Love* depends on this but does not emerge automatically from it. What distinguishes this is not the presence of positive feeling, but the capacity to sustain contact—with oneself and with the other—without immediate recourse to defense. This contact may remain partial, qualified, or uneven, but no longer collapses as quickly under pressure.

Jessica Benjamin's (2018) formulation of mutual recognition is useful here as a structural reference point, rather than an achieved state. The capacity to register the other as separate, while remaining in contact with one's own experience, requires a degree of internal stability that is not available earlier in the process. *Love*, as positioned in the model, reflects movement toward this capacity, though it may appear in limited or unstable forms.

Klein's (1957/1975) account of reparation also informs this placement, particularly in relation to the endurance of the object. If *Gratitude* allows for the internalization of what is experienced as good, *Love* involves the ability to maintain that relation in the presence of ambivalence, frustration, or conflict. The object is no longer immediately lost or attacked when tension arises, though it may still be subjected to distortion or control.

*Love* does not consolidate what precedes it, nor does it resolve earlier tensions. It introduces a different relation to them. What becomes possible is not coherence in a final sense, but a capacity to remain in contact—without immediate withdrawal, collapse, or reorganization. The experience may be brief, uneven, or difficult to sustain, but it reflects a change in how both self and other can be held.

## Concluding Reflections

*Love*, as it appears in the surrender process, does not announce itself as a resolution or arrival. It emerges in how experience is held differently—less immediately defended against, less quickly reorganized. What shifts is not the presence of feeling, but the conditions under which it can remain.

What characterizes this is not stability, but a change in tolerance. Contact no longer collapses in the same way, even if it cannot yet be sustained. Experience may still be qualified, dispersed, or brought under control, but is not immediately foreclosed. Something is permitted to register before it is altered or lost.

This shift does not produce coherence in any final sense. It introduces a different relation to incoherence. Ambivalence, dependency, and recognition can begin to coexist without requiring immediate resolution. The experience remains uneven, and often difficult to hold, but it no longer necessitates the same degree of withdrawal or attack.

Winnicott's (1958) formulation of the capacity to be alone offers a useful frame here, not as a conclusion, but as a condition that begins to register. The presence of the other is not consistently internalized, nor reliably available, but it is no longer entirely absent. It may appear intermittently, and under specific conditions, as something that can be referred to without being immediately lost.

What characterizes this is not stability but a change in tolerance. Contact no longer collapses in the same way, even if it cannot yet be sustained. Experience may still be qualified, dispersed, or brought under control, but is not immediately foreclosed. Something is permitted to register before it is altered or lost.

In this sense, *Love* reflects a shift in what can be endured: contact that can be approached without immediate defense, recognition that can persist without immediate collapse, and the possibility—however limited—that something of the self or the other can be held without being evacuated or controlled.

# 26 Wisdom

*Wisdom* occupies a later position in the surrender process, not as a final state, but as a shift in how experience is known and lived. It reflects a form of knowing that does not rely on abstraction or distance but emerges through sustained contact with one's internal life. In psychoanalytic terms, it is less a cognitive achievement than a way of holding experience—one that develops through repeated encounters with what could not previously be borne.

This becomes apparent when knowing is no longer separate from experience—when changes are carried in how one lives, feels, and relates, rather than observed from a distance. It reflects a change in how the self encounters itself: not through rigid defense or isolated insight, but through an increasing capacity to remain with internal experience without immediate reorganization. This capacity does not arrive at once. It develops over time, through repeated exposures to affective strain, containment, and recognition. What emerges is not certainty, but a different order of clarity—one that is grounded, provisional, and responsive to complexity.

Gendlin (1981, 1997) and Greenberg (1987) distinguish between conceptual knowledge and a felt sense of knowing—what Gendlin describes as a "felt shift," a bodily recognition that something has moved or realigned. This form of knowing is not simply reflective; it is lived. It appears as a convergence of affect and thought, where experience is not only understood but carried.

Winnicott (1949/1975) observed that

> All individuals are really trying to find a new birth in which the line of their own life will not be disturbed by a quantity of reacting greater than that which can be experienced without a loss of the sense of continuity of personal existence.
>
> (p. 188)

This formulation situates surrender within the limits of what can be experienced without disruption. Surrender does not proceed through collapse but through conditions in which experience can be taken in without

DOI: 10.4324/9781003795803-31

overwhelming the continuity of the self. When pressure exceeds this threshold, defensive organization or dissociation reasserts itself. In this sense, what appears here as wisdom is not the resolution of conflict, but a change in what can be borne: greater tolerance for complexity, sustained affective contact under strain, and the capacity to metabolize experience without immediate fragmentation.

## Jerome

Jerome sat back in the chair, legs crossed, his hands resting open for once—not clenched, not calculating. He looked at them briefly, as if noticing the position.

"It's strange," he said. "I don't feel like I'm fighting in the same way."

I didn't respond.

"I used to think life was about keeping the edges clean—showing up sharp, composed." A faint tightening at the corner of his mouth. "No room for... slippage."

He adjusted his cuff, then stopped, leaving it slightly uneven.

"But lately..." He paused. "It's harder to sustain that." A small exhale. "Not because I can't. I just—" He stopped again. "I don't see the point in the same way."

He glanced toward the window, then back.

"I've been noticing how much effort it took. The way I kept everything... contained." A slight emphasis on the word, as if testing it. "And now when I look at it, it feels..." He searched. "Not wrong. Just... unnecessary."

A pause.

"I'm not saying I've resolved anything," he added. "I don't think that's how this works." A brief glance toward me. "But I don't feel the same pressure to correct myself all the time."

He leaned back, then forward again, forearms resting on his knees.

"Parts of me I would've moved to fix—or at least reframe—they're still there. I just don't... go after them in the same way."

Silence held.

I said, "You're not intervening as quickly."

He gave a low, almost surprised laugh.

"That's one way to put it." He nodded once. "Yeah."

He sat with that for a moment, then added:

"And I'm not entirely comfortable with that." A slight narrowing of his eyes. "There's a part of me that still thinks something's being missed. Or neglected."

He paused again.

"But it's not as loud."

His hands shifted slightly in his lap, then settled again.

"I don't think this came from one thing," he continued. "It's more... cumulative." A small gesture with his hand, as if layering something.

"Moments that didn't get resolved. Things I didn't push through or clean up."

He looked down briefly.

"And somehow that's stayed." A pause. "Not as a conclusion. Just... there."

I said, "You didn't finish it."

He looked up, a slight pause.

"No," he said. "I didn't." A faint shift in his expression. "Which would usually bother me more."

Silence held.

"I didn't expect that," he added. "That something like that could hold without being finalized."

He leaned back again, more slowly this time.

"Usually I'd want to name it more precisely," he said. "Make sure I wasn't overstating it." A brief glance toward me. "I'm aware I'm not doing that right now."

The room held there.

After a while, he stood, adjusting his sleeve again—more out of habit than necessity.

At the door, he paused briefly, then left.

A change is evident in Jerome's relation to his internal experience, but it does not replace his reliance on mastery. The impulse to define, qualify, and organize remains present, though it is no longer immediate. Experience can be allowed to persist without being fully resolved, but not without tension. What appears is not consolidation, but a partial suspension of control—limited, provisional, and dependent on continued conditions that support it.

## Bill

Bill came in for his session on a rainy Wednesday, still wearing his work boots. He sat down with the usual thud, leaned forward, and rested his forearms on his knees. A faint smell of oil followed him in.

"So I was at Ronny's this weekend," he said. "He was changing the brake pads on his truck. Asked if I'd give him a hand."

I nodded.

There was a long pause. Bill scratched at a grease mark on his thumbnail, picking at it with more focus than it required.

"We didn't talk much. Just worked." He shrugged. "You know how it is."

Another pause.

"But at one point he leaned back—like this—" He shifted slightly, demonstrating, then stopped halfway through the motion. "Wiped his hands on a rag. Just sat there a second, looking out at the yard."

He looked down again.

"And he goes, 'This is the life.'"

A brief silence.

Bill's mouth twitched, almost a smile.

"I've known him twenty years," he said. "Same guy. Same place." He shook his head once. "He's got less than I do. Works longer hours."

He paused.

"But it didn't sound like bullshit."

He glanced up, then away.

"He meant it."

I said, "Sounds like he was content in a way that caught you off guard."

Bill nodded once.

"Yeah."

The room settled again.

"I don't know why that stuck with me," he said. "It just... did."

His fingers pressed into his palm, then released.

"It made me think—" He stopped. "I don't know. Like maybe..." He let the sentence drop.

I didn't speak.

He shifted in the chair.

"I'm not saying I've been doing it wrong," he added. "I mean, things are fine." A small nod, as if confirming it to himself.

Another pause.

"But there was something in the way he said it." He frowned slightly. "Like he wasn't trying to convince anybody."

Silence.

"Like he already knew," he said. Then, after a beat: "Or didn't need to."

He sat back a little, not fully, just enough to ease the pressure in his posture.

"I don't know what that is," he added. "Or what you do with it."

I said, "You noticed it."

Bill nodded again.

"Yeah."

He didn't elaborate.

The silence stretched, but he didn't move to fill it. His foot shifted once against the floor, then stilled.

After a moment, he leaned forward again, forearms returning to his knees.

"That's it," he said.

He stayed there a second longer, then looked toward the door.

A shift occurs in Bill's relation to experience, but it does not organize into reflection. What registers is external and concrete—located in the observation of another rather than within himself. The experience is noted but not elaborated. It remains unformulated, carried without symbolic development. What becomes possible is limited to recognition without integration, and a brief suspension of his usual focus on action or correction.

## What It Asks of the Therapist

*Wisdom* asks the therapist to sustain a stance of openness—one that allows the patient's emerging understanding to unfold without interruption or premature framing. At this point in the surrender process, meaning is no longer assembled in fragments but begins to hold together in a lived way. The therapist's role is not to affirm or explain, but to register what has changed: a different rhythm in the patient's speech, a reduced need to defend or perform, a steadiness that was not previously available.

With Jerome, the therapist may notice a subtle internal quieting—an absence of the usual pressure to track, interpret, or maintain the frame. As Jerome sits with his hands open, no longer clenched, something in the therapist's own stance may ease in response. There is less urgency to do anything with what is being said. When Jerome speaks of "not fighting anymore," or of no longer hating the parts of himself he once tried to fix, the therapist may feel both moved and, in a certain way, less central. Not dismissed but no longer required in the same way. The countertransference reflects this shift: a sense of stillness, a release of effort, and a recognition that the work is being carried from within the patient rather than organized from outside.

Bill's session may evoke something different. As he describes Ronny's quiet contentment, the therapist may feel a pull toward completion—a wish to help him put language to what he is circling. His comment—"Like he knew something I didn't. Or maybe I did, once"—lands with weight but does not develop further. The therapist may notice an urge to gather the moment, to give it shape. This, too, belongs to the countertransference: a desire for the experience to resolve into something clearer than it is. What is required instead is restraint—not withdrawal, but the maintenance of a boundary around something still forming. The therapist's softness can meet Bill's without moving ahead of it.

These differences point to the therapist's task: to use countertransference as a way of reading the process rather than directing it. Feelings of stillness, pressure, reverence, or longing are not signals to act, but forms through which the unfolding of the work registers in the analytic field. *Wisdom*, when it appears, may bring relief, stillness, uncertainty, or even unease. These responses are sustained as part of the process, without being organized too quickly into meaning or action.

*Wisdom* is not always spoken. It may show itself in a change in posture, a slowing of speech, or a shift in what holds importance. To name it too early risks replacing it with explanation. The therapist's experience must be held carefully—not dismissed but not imposed.

In this sense, the therapist becomes responsible for preserving the conditions in which something can continue to develop. What is asked is not intervention, but steadiness: an ability to remain present without pressing the moment into clarity. When wisdom emerges, it is often the result of many prior movements—ruptures, recognitions, and returns. To meet it without disrupting it, and to allow it to remain as it is, is one of the more demanding aspects of the work.

## Justification for the Placement of this Configuration

*Wisdom* emerges as a later integrative phase within the surrender process, following the relational and affective openings of *Shift, Gratitude*, and *Love*. It reflects a point at which the accumulated experiences of surrender—across vulnerability, insight, and change—begin to settle into something more stable. This does not bring the process to a close. Instead, it introduces a form of internal consolidation: what has been encountered can now be carried with less disruption.

The individual's relation to their own history comes under change. Experience is no longer approached solely through the lens of injury or adaptation but is held within a wider frame in which multiple meanings can coexist. Conflict does not resolve and uncertainty is not eliminated. Both remain in contact without the same immediate return to defensive organization. What changes is not the presence of difficulty, but the conditions under which it is borne.

*Wisdom* reflects a change in the quality of knowing itself. This form of knowing is bodily and affective—something registered rather than constructed, arising within the felt continuity of experience rather than imposed upon it Gendlin (1997) and Greenberg (1987). It does not depend on articulation in order to be trusted, nor does it require immediate translation into thought. What distinguishes this from earlier moments is not the arrival of new insight, but the way insight is lived, carried, and returned to over time, as part of an ongoing relation rather than a discrete event.

At the same time, *Wisdom* does not stabilize the process once and for all. Later configurations—*Revealing, Unconcealment, Dynamic Flow, Repetition*, and *Nameless Dread*—may reopen disorientation, grief, or fragmentation, returning the individual to forms of experience that are not fully assimilated. What is made available is not protection from those movements but a different mode of encounter with them, in which contact can be sustained without the same immediate need for defense or withdrawal. With something more established internally, the individual is less readily overtaken by what emerges and more able to remain in relation to it as it unfolds. In this sense, *Wisdom* extends the process rather than completing it, reflecting a readiness to continue within it rather than to move beyond it.

## Concluding Reflections

*Wisdom* does not arrive as a conclusion. It appears more quietly, as a shift in how experience is held. What has been separate begins, at times, to sit together without immediate correction. There is less urgency to resolve, less pressure to organize. Something steadier becomes available—not fixed, but usable.

This does not remove conflict. Contradiction remains, as does uncertainty. What changes is the individual's capacity to stay in contact with both. Where there was once collapse or avoidance, there may now be a pause, or a willingness to remain. The difference is often subtle, but it alters what can be lived with.

*Wisdom* also changes the way experience is approached. Pain is no longer encountered only as something to be eliminated or explained, but as something that can be stayed with. This does not make it easier. It makes it more possible. The internal space around experience widens, even when the experience itself does not.

These shifts do not appear uniformly. For some, they take the form of something that has begun to hold together—less driven, less organized around proving. For others, they emerge as something more limited: a moment of recognition that does not yet reorganize the self but is allowed to register without being dismissed or forced into clarity. What joins these experiences is not mastery but a change in how one relates to what arises—a loosening of the need to finalize what is still in motion.

For the therapist, these moments are rarely marked by intensity. They tend to arrive without emphasis—through a change in tone, pacing, or presence. The task is not to name them or extend them, but to remain with them as they are. Any attempt to fix or define them too quickly risks replacing the experience with explanation.

*Wisdom* does not complete the work. It alters the conditions under which the work continues. What becomes possible is not resolution, but a different relationship to what unfolds—one that can hold, return, and remain in contact without needing to finalize what is still unfolding.

# 27 Revealing

As the fifth configuration in Releasement Level C—corresponding to the body's circulatory and endocrine systems—*Revealing* reflects a change in the surrender process. The patient's inner life comes into view with greater ease, not as something produced through effort, but as something that begins to show itself. Articulation no longer functions primarily as a means of control or explanation; it becomes a medium through which experience unfolds in real time. What emerges is not simply insight, but something that can be spoken as it is being lived—an experience that carries its own coherence without requiring construction in advance.[1]

Clinically, this configuration reflects not the initial formation of symbols, but their fuller use within the analytic situation. Material that had previously been present but difficult to access or sustain begins to move with greater continuity in speech and thought. What distinguishes *Revealing* is not the intensity of discovery—as in earlier configurations—but the patient's increasing capacity to remain with what is emerging and give it form as it develops. The symbolic capacities established earlier are now held within a relational frame that supports this ongoing articulation. As Bollas (1981) suggests, aspects of the self must first be allowed to emerge and take shape before they can be understood.[2] In this configuration, that emergence becomes more continuous: what had been fragmented or held back can now be spoken, felt, and taken in as one's own.

Here, the analytic work takes on a different rhythm. Meaning and affect begin to circulate more freely, without the same interruptions or need for control. What comes forward is not forced or searched for. It arrives in the course of speaking, sometimes unexpectedly, but with a sense of recognition that does not require immediate explanation. What had been difficult to hold together can now be carried in a more sustained way.

Earlier forms of exposure may occur without this continuity—material may be spoken but not sustained, expressed without being taken up as part of the self.

What emerges here remains within the patient's capacity to hold and articulate it as it develops. When that capacity is exceeded—when what comes forward can no longer be carried in language without strain or disruption—the process moves beyond this configuration.

DOI: 10.4324/9781003795803-32

## Winston

Winston sat down and looked at the floor.

"I don't know what we're doing anymore," he said. "Not in a bad way. Just... I used to come in here ready to say something clever, or weird, or angry." He exhaled. "Now I don't want to perform. I want to... stay in it a little longer."

I let that sit.

"That's different," I said.

He nodded, still looking down.

"I've been thinking about this memory," he went on. "I've never said it out loud."

A pause.

"My dad took me fishing once," he said. "Just once."

A pause.

"He didn't really do things like that. He was... busy." A faint, almost apologetic shrug.

"We were on this small boat. I remember trying to do everything right." He glanced down. "I dropped the pole in the water."

He exhaled through his nose.

"He snapped. Not loud, just—sharp." A quick motion with his hand. "Like I'd ruined something."

Winston paused.

"And then, a second later, he laughed. Like it didn't matter. Like I was supposed to laugh too."

He looked up briefly.

"I didn't know which one was real."

A beat.

"If I'd messed up... or if it was nothing."

He shook his head slightly.

"I still don't."

I didn't respond.

He sat with it.

"I think I used to try to figure it out," he said. "Like, what it meant. What it said about him. About me." He shrugged. "Now I don't know. I just... wanted to say it."

"It stayed with you," I said.

"Yeah." A small nod. "More than I realized."

The room went quiet again, but he didn't move away from it.

Later in the session, he said, "It's strange—I used to leave here with ten different ideas." A faint smile. "Now I just leave... quieter."

I glanced toward him.

"Not empty," he added. "Just... not trying to solve it."

Winston's material emerges with greater continuity, but without a corresponding need to organize or resolve it. The memory is spoken, held, and allowed to remain ambiguous. What changes is not the content itself, but his relation to it: he stays with the experience as it unfolds, rather than moving to interpret or manage it. Articulation becomes possible without closure. The process remains active but not directed toward conclusion.

## Gabriella

Gabriella, a retired teacher, had spent most of her adult life speaking with poise and restraint. Even after years of therapy, her words often arrived carefully arranged, as though each sentence had been checked before it was allowed out.

That day, she sat back slightly, as if noticing something as she spoke.

"I used to organize everything I said in here," she said. "Like I was preparing something." A small smile. "Making sure it made sense before I said it."

She paused.

"And now..." She exhaled. "I'm not doing that."

I waited.

"It's strange," she continued. "I'll start a sentence and I don't actually know where it's going." A faint laugh, not quite comfortable. "And I'm letting it happen."

I said, "You're not correcting it as you go."

She shook her head.

"No. Or... less." She glanced down, then back up. "It feels a little exposed. But also—" She stopped, searching. "Clearer, maybe. Even if it's not finished."

A pause.

"I'm saying things I didn't think I could say," she added. "Not because I didn't have the words. I just..." She hesitated. "Wouldn't let them line up that way."

I didn't respond.

She sat with that.

"My mother didn't say much," she went on, more slowly now. "But you always knew what not to say." A brief tightening in her expression. "You could feel it."

She glanced toward me.

"So I got very good at... adjusting." A small hand movement, as if smoothing something out. "Even here."

Another pause.

"And now I'm not doing that in the same way." She frowned slightly. "Or I am—but I notice it. And sometimes I don't follow it."

She let that sit.

"I don't think I'm less careful," she said after a moment. "I think I'm... staying with myself more while I'm talking."

I said, "You're not leaving the experience as quickly."

She nodded.

"Yes." A quieter tone. "That's what it feels like."

Silence settled, but she didn't rush to fill it.

After a moment, she added, almost to herself, "It's not as polished. But it feels more like mine."

Gabriella's speech becomes less organized in advance and more shaped in the moment. What changes is not the content alone, but her relation to expression itself: she remains with her experience as it forms, rather than editing it before it is spoken. Language, affect, and memory begin to move together with less interruption. This does not eliminate self-monitoring but loosens its dominance. Articulation becomes possible without prior structuring, and what emerges is taken up as her own while still in development.

## What It Asks of the Therapist

*Revealing* asks the therapist to offer a presence that is attuned yet restrained, responsive yet non-intrusive, capable of registering what emerges without moving to define it. Rather than guiding or interpreting, the therapist sustains a posture that allows the patient's emerging coherence to unfold without interruption, within a frame that can bear articulation as it takes shape. What appears here is often not new material, but a different relation to saying—one that requires a frame capable of holding articulation as it develops, rather than organizing it prematurely.

With Winston, something in the room shifts from effort to contact. After many sessions marked by deflection, cleverness, or distance, his speech begins to carry affect without performance. As he speaks about the memory with his father, the therapist may feel a quiet settling—alongside a subtle pull to name the moment, to deepen it, or to secure its meaning. There may also be a transference shift: Winston is no longer relating through performance or provocation but allowing himself to be seen in a more direct way, without testing or managing the therapist's response. The countertransference here includes both relief and a kind of tenderness, which can easily become an urge to respond more than is needed. A simple reflection—"It mattered"—is sufficient. It marks the moment without organizing it, allowing the experience to remain his.

With Gabriella, the shift appears in the movement of language itself. As her speech becomes less arranged and more immediate, the relational field opens. The therapist may feel more included, less held at a distance by her precision. At the same time, this can bring a subtle pull to align with her—to stay with what is articulate, coherent, and easy to receive. This is where the risk of collusion emerges: not as overt agreement, but as a quiet tendency to follow her lead too closely, allowing her longstanding adaptation to remain intact. Her transference may carry an expectation that she will be received when she is composed, thoughtful, and careful; the therapist may feel invited into that arrangement. What is required is a response that stays with her experience without reinforcing that pattern. When the therapist reflects—

"It's like you're letting the words find you"—the aim is not to affirm her performance, but to remain alongside her as something less managed comes into form.

In both cases, the task is not to facilitate insight, but to hold the conditions in which expression becomes increasingly owned. The countertransference may include relief, warmth, hope, or a wish to consolidate what is emerging. These are not errors, but signals of proximity to something real. The discipline lies in not acting on them too quickly.

What is asked is a particular kind of restraint—not silence, but a refusal to get ahead of the patient's experience. Interpretation, if it comes too soon, risks replacing what is forming with something already known. The therapist must stay close without shaping, responsive without directing.

In these moments, transference comes under a different organization, no longer oriented primarily toward managing the therapist but toward using the analytic space more directly. The patient is less concerned with how they are received and more engaged in articulating what is internally present as it takes form in language. The therapist's role is to meet this change without amplifying it, allowing the patient's language to carry its own authority within the relational field.

*Revealing* does not call for increased activity on the part of the therapist. It requires less intervention, but with greater precision of attention. To listen without organizing. To respond without closing. To recognize that what is emerging is already in motion—and that the work, at this point, lies in allowing it to continue without interruption or premature structuring.

## Justification for the Placement of this Configuration

*Revealing* emerges as a later configuration in the surrender process, made possible by the conditions established in *Gratitude, Love,* and *Wisdom.* These earlier configurations do not simply produce insight; they establish the internal and relational stability within which experience can be felt, held, and symbolized without collapse or defensive retreat. By this point, the patient is no longer organizing their inner life in response to threat or evaluation. Something has settled sufficiently for experience to begin taking form on its own, without being directed or secured in advance.

What distinguishes *Revealing* is not the appearance of new material, but a change in how material comes into language. The patient is no longer working to understand, clarify, or present their experience. Instead, they begin to speak from within it, with language emerging in continuity with feeling rather than in response to it. Language becomes less strategic and more contiguous with experience—less an attempt to arrive somewhere and more a way of remaining in contact with what is already present.

Clinically, *Revealing* sits at a critical juncture. It follows *Wisdom,* where a degree of internal coherence and reflective capacity has been established, and it precedes *Unconcealment,* where that coherence may be strained or disrupted by what emerges next. Its placement here is not incidental. It functions as a point of circulation: affect, meaning, and symbolization begin to move together with greater continuity, allowing experience to be expressed without fragmenting or becoming overdetermined.

Without this phase, the patient may encounter *Unconcealment* either defensively or prematurely—flooded by what cannot yet be articulated or forced back into interpretation as a form of control. *Revealing* provides something more specific than 'integration': it establishes the capacity to remain in contact with emerging experience as it takes shape, without needing to resolve it.

In this sense, the significance here lies not in what is said, but in how it is carried in the act of saying. The patient is no longer only processing internally; they are beginning to live in language differently—speaking in a way that is less organized around outcome and more grounded in presence. This development, subtle as it may appear, reflects a change in how experience is held and expressed within the analytic field. It allows what has been metabolized to enter shared space without distortion and prepares the psyche for the more destabilizing movements that follow.

## Concluding Reflections

*Revealing* marks a shift in the analytic process that is easy to overlook precisely because it does not announce itself. There is no rupture, no dramatic insight—only a change in how experience moves. What has been held internally begins to find expression without being forced, shaped, or defended against. Speech becomes less an act of construction and more an extension of contact.

This is not a return to content, but a change in relation to it. The patient is no longer trying to decipher what something means or secure it through explanation. Instead, experience is allowed to unfold in language as it is lived. What emerges may be incomplete, uncertain, or unformulated—but it is no longer avoided. It is carried forward.

Coltart's (1985) emphasis on remaining open to what cannot be anticipated is particularly relevant here. The work depends on a capacity—on both sides—to remain in contact with what has not yet taken shape, without moving to organize or secure it prematurely. This often entails a loosening of the usual reliance on thought as a structuring force within the analytic process. Not the absence of thinking, but a willingness to let it follow rather than lead, emerging in response to experience rather than determining it in advance.

For the therapist, this shifts the task in a subtle but significant way. The pressure to interpret diminishes, but another demand takes its place: to remain with what is forming without organizing it prematurely. The work becomes one of accompaniment rather than clarification—of allowing language to develop from within the patient's experience rather than imposing coherence from outside it.

*Revealing* does not resolve the process of surrender. It brings the patient into more direct contact with it, as what has been metabolized can now be spoken while what has not begins to press forward. In this way, the configuration holds both consolidation and risk. It stabilizes expression while opening the possibility of encountering what remains unintegrated within the emerging field of experience.

What matters here is not the completeness of what is said, but the fact that it can be said at all—without performance, without evasion, and without the need to arrive at a conclusion. In that shift, something essential changes. The patient is no longer relating to their experience from a distance. They are speaking from within it.

## Notes

1 A form of revealing appears earlier, particularly in *Gratitude*, where aspects of the self come forward without being directly intended. Exposure occurs indirectly, shaped by the presence of trust and containment, and may not yet be fully recognized, symbolized, or taken up by the patient within the analytic process.

In the present configuration, this process undergoes a change. *Revealing* becomes more participatory: the patient begins, at times, to remain with what is emerging and to give it form in speech as it unfolds. This does not reflect full intention or control, but a greater involvement in the act of expression—an increased willingness to stay with, elaborate, and articulate one's experience as it takes shape within the relational frame.

2 Bollas' observation points to the stance required here. Rather than moving quickly to interpret or organize what emerges, the analyst allows the material to take shape within the relational frame, where it can develop without premature structuring. The task becomes less a matter of uncovering hidden meaning than of remaining with what is forming, so that it can be spoken, felt, and gradually taken up by the patient as their own within the analytic process.

# 28 Unconcealment

*Unconcealment* reflects a structural change in the surrender process—not a moment of revelation, but a loosening of the need to keep certain aspects of experience hidden. The preceding configuration, *Revealing,* allows experience to come into language with greater continuity and presence. *Unconcealment* moves further: the patient begins to relinquish reliance on distortion as a way of organizing what can be known, as material comes forward that is less mediated by prior defensive structure.

This is not a configuration of discovery, but of release. Defensive arrangements that once shaped perception and meaning begin to lose their necessity as organizing principles. The patient no longer sustains the version of reality that once made experience bearable. What emerges is often not new. Long-standing patterns, memories, or recognitions come into view with a different quality—less charged, less resisted, less subject to alteration. The change lies not in what is seen, but in the absence of the effort required to keep it out of awareness.

Clinically, this may appear as a quiet reduction in rationalization, projection, or narrative control. The patient becomes less invested in explaining, justifying, or arranging their experience. Instead, they begin to remain in contact with aspects of themselves that had previously required denial or distance. Affect tends to settle into something more proportionate—not because it is diminished, but because it is no longer being managed through distortion. Interpretation becomes less central. There is more room for experience to register as it is.

Philosophically, this configuration resonates with Heidegger's notion of *aletheia*—unconcealment—not as the arrival of a correct account, but as the coming-into-presence of what had been obscured (Heidegger, 1962). In this sense, nothing is 'uncovered' in the conventional way. Rather, what had been held out of view—through necessity, not choice—comes to stand in the open within experience. The patient does not acquire new knowledge so much as regain access to what had long been inaccessible, now encountered without the same conditions of exclusion.

What changes is the patient's relation to their own mind. Experience no longer has to be shaped in order to be tolerated. What once required

DOI: 10.4324/9781003795803-33

disavowal can be held in awareness without immediate retreat. The movement is gradual and often understated. Illusion does not collapse dramatically; it loses its function. In its place, a different kind of coherence begins to take hold—one that does not depend on keeping certain truths out of sight.

## Jerome

Jerome sat back, one ankle resting over his knee, fingers loosely interlaced. He was quiet longer than usual.

"When I was about eight," he said finally, "I drew this picture. A robot with a cape." A faint breath, almost dismissive. "I remember showing it to someone at school. I don't even remember who now."

He paused.

"They looked at it for a second. Didn't really react. Just sort of... moved on."

Another pause. His tone stayed even, but something in it had thinned.

"I don't think it registered as anything at the time," he said. "But I must have taken something from it." A slight shift in posture. "That it wasn't... necessary."

I said, "Something about not making it matter."

He nodded once.

"I got very good at that," he said. "At making sure it didn't." A small exhale. "At not putting myself in a position where it would."

The room settled.

A few minutes later, he spoke again, more quietly.

"It's strange," he said. "Even saying that now—I can feel it doesn't quite hold." He frowned slightly, as if tracking something internally. "It didn't go anywhere." A brief pause. "I just kept it contained."

I said, "It's still there."

A faint, almost wry smile.

"Yeah. I used to think my competence was just who I was." He looked off for a moment. "Now it feels more like something I built. Something that had to be there."

Silence again.

"It worked," he added. "It still works." A longer pause. "But it's not all of it."

The room held there—without pressure, without movement.

Near the end of the session, he said, almost under his breath, "I think I've been telling myself a story about not needing much."

He didn't look up.

"I'm just... not sure I believe it the same way anymore."

## Gabriella

"And then he didn't even ask how I was," Gabriella said. "After everything. It's like—I could have been anyone."

She paused, but didn't stop.

"I keep going back to it," she said. "The last thing I said to him. The way I said it." A small shake of her head. "I can hear it. I can almost fix it."

I listened.

"Like—maybe I came on too strong," she said. "Or I said something that put him off." A brief pause. "Or he just... wasn't able to stay with it."

She frowned slightly.

"I can usually land on something."

She looked down.

"But this one doesn't."

Silence.

"I keep replaying it," she said. "Trying to understand why he just... shut down." A faint tightening in her voice. "And I can't get it to line up."

I said, "It's not coming together in the way it usually does."

She shook her head.

"No." A longer pause. "It usually does."

The room shifted.

"I can feel myself trying to do the thing I always do," she said. "Make it make sense. Put it somewhere." She looked up briefly. "So I know where I stand."

I didn't respond.

"But when I go back to it..." she said, slower now, "there's just that moment where he pulls away. And I can't... get past it." A pause. "I don't know what I did."

Silence settled.

"And I keep trying to turn it into something familiar," she said. "Like—I was too much, or not enough, or he couldn't handle it. Something." A faint, almost frustrated breath. "But none of it sticks."

I said, "You can't settle on a version of it."

She nodded.

"No." A pause. "It won't stay still."

The room held.

"I think I've always been able to make these things make sense," she said. "Even when they hurt." She looked down again. "This just... hurts."

I waited.

After a while, she said, quietly, "I don't know what to do with that."

I said, "You're not trying to fix it right now."

She shook her head.

"No." A pause. "I don't think I can."

Silence held.

"That's different," she said.

## What It Asks of the Therapist

In *Unconcealment*, the therapist is asked to hold a particular tension: to remain fully present while not giving premature shape to what is emerging, even as the pressure to do so increases. This is not a configuration that calls for interpretation or clarification, but for the capacity to stay with experience as it loses its usual organization within the analytic field. The patient may still attempt to make sense of what is happening, but the familiar pathways no longer resolve. What once settled into meaning no longer does, and experience remains in a state that resists immediate formulation.

The pressure on the therapist arises precisely here. There can be a strong pull to restore coherence—to help the patient arrive at an understanding, to locate cause, or to offer a formulation that stabilizes the moment. But this risks reconstituting the very structure that is beginning to loosen. The work is not to organize the experience, but to remain with it as it fails to take form.

As Thomas H. Ogden (1994) observes, "The analyst must resist the temptation to define what is occurring too quickly or too completely. The analyst's task is to help create the conditions in which something new and unexpected can come into being" (p. 9). In this configuration, containment is not only a matter of safety, but of sustaining contact with what cannot yet be thought, where experience remains present without consolidation into meaning. The patient may return to familiar material, but it is no longer metabolized in the same way. The narrative remains, but its organizing function has weakened, no longer securing coherence in the way it once did. The therapist may find themselves responding not only to what is said, but to a change in its weight—something less resolved, less usable, and less available for immediate integration.

This shift is often registered first in the countertransference. With Gabriella, the therapist may feel disoriented as her usual fluency no longer organizes the room, alongside a pull to restore continuity—to help her find her footing through language. At the same time, something less familiar emerges: the sense that the structure of her story no longer holds. In the transference, this may take the form of an unspoken appeal to be brought back into coherence—to have the experience made sense of so that she can again occupy a recognizable position.

With Jerome, the countertransference may include a quiet respect for his relinquishment of control, alongside a sense of loss as a long-standing mode of self-definition falls away. There may be a pull to acknowledge or affirm what is being given up—to recognize the significance of the shift. But even this can move too quickly to stabilize the experience. In the transference, the therapist may be positioned as the one who can confirm who Jerome is now that the performance has loosened.

In both cases, the task is to resist occupying that position. The patient is not only revealing something—they are losing the frame that made their experience intelligible. To name this too soon, or to consolidate it into meaning, risks converting a structural change into a moment of insight. The therapist must instead tolerate the absence of resolution, allowing the patient's contact with what is unformulated to continue without being gathered into coherence.

*Unconcealment* is not the arrival of clarity, but the failure of what once produced it. What it asks of the therapist is the capacity to remain with that failure—without repairing it, and without turning away.

## Justification for the Placement of this Configuration

*Unconcealment* emerges only after the patient has developed the capacity to encounter previously disavowed experience and to take it up as their own within the analytic process. In earlier configurations, what was split off becomes available, and the patient can begin to articulate it in language. But this articulation remains organized, shaped by forms that allow it to be held, understood, and, to some extent, managed within existing structures of meaning.

What changes here is not the content, but the function of that organization. The patient no longer relies on explanation to maintain contact with themselves. The familiar movement toward coherence continues, but it no longer resolves. What had once stabilized experience begins to lose its necessity.

This shift places *Unconcealment* after *Revealing* and *Wisdom*, but before any sustained movement can occur. As long as experience must be shaped in order to be tolerated, it remains partially governed. The patient may return repeatedly to insight, but insight continues to serve a structuring function.

Only when that structuring begins to fall away does a different kind of movement become possible. Without *Unconcealment*, subsequent change is reorganized around what is already known. With it, experience is no longer required to arrive in a form that can be secured in advance.

*Unconcealment* belongs here because it marks the point at which the patient can remain in contact with experience without first converting it into something that can be held in place.

## Concluding Reflections

*Unconcealment* can resemble insight, but it does not function as one. Nothing new is discovered, and nothing is clarified in the usual sense. What changes is the need to arrive at clarity at all.

The patient continues to speak, but speech no longer organizes the experience in the same way. What had previously been used to secure coherence begins to fall out of use. The experience does not resolve and is no longer required to.

This alters the conditions under which further change can occur. As long as experience must be rendered intelligible in order to be tolerated, it remains partially shaped in advance. When that requirement loosens, something else becomes possible—not as an achievement, but as a consequence of no longer needing to hold experience in place.

What follows is not an expansion, but a different relation to what is already present. Experience is no longer approached through the demand that it be understood before it can be lived.

# 29 Dynamic Flow

*Dynamic Flow* begins to register when the patient no longer needs to gather themselves in the same way. It follows *Unconcealment* and precedes *Repetition* and *A Nameless Dread,* marking a point at which experience can move without being secured in advance. What had previously required effort—holding onto a line of thought, managing affect as it arises, keeping experience within a tolerable frame—no longer demands the same degree of intervention. The patient still speaks, still thinks, still reflects, but the activity is less organized around securing position.

This shift is not experienced as a new state, nor as an increase in coherence. Rather, the patient finds themselves continuing where they would previously have stopped. A thought can give way to another without being resolved. An affect can emerge, intensify, and recede without being shaped into something usable. What might once have been interrupted—by explanation, by self-correction, by the need to understand—now proceeds.

There is often a change in how the patient inhabits the session. They may follow an association further than before, without returning to clarify it. They may speak from within an experience rather than about it, without translating it into meaning. Contradictory positions can appear in proximity without urgency to reconcile them. The mind does not lose structure, but it is no longer required to assert it in the same way.

Because experience is no longer required to settle into coherence, it can also return differently. Material that has already been encountered may reappear without the same pressure to organize or master it, setting the conditions for what will later be taken up more directly in *Repetition*. At the same time, as the structures that once held experience in place become less active, there are moments when nothing replaces them. The continuity that has begun to form does not yet provide stability, and the patient may come into contact with states that are more diffuse, less bounded, and harder to locate—conditions that deepen in *A Nameless Dread*.

In this sense, *Dynamic Flow* reflects a change in how psychic activity proceeds. Bion's formulation of negative capability (1970) becomes more available—not as an attitude to be adopted, but as a condition that is no longer resisted. Ferro's description of a polyphonic field is also relevant

DOI: 10.4324/9781003795803-34

here, in that multiple strands of experience can unfold without requiring reduction to a single line of meaning. These are not new capacities so much as previously constrained ones that are no longer being held in check.

*Dynamic Flow* does not mark an arrival. It marks the point at which movement can be sustained without needing to be organized in advance.

## Bill

Bill talked about his truck, about the price of lumber, about how drywall used to be thicker. He would move from one thing to the next without pausing long enough for anything to gather.

There were weeks, though, when the pacing changed. He had started walking again. Not far—just down to the hardware store and back. He didn't present it as a decision. It came up the same way everything else did.

"Been going down there in the mornings," he said. "Just to get out."

He didn't elaborate.

One afternoon, he mentioned that a man he had served with had died by suicide. He said it plainly, then went quiet. The silence held longer than usual.

"I used to think he had it more together than me," he said. A pause. "Turns out maybe I wasn't the only one who didn't know what to do."

I waited.

He didn't move to explain it. He didn't shift away.

"He had a house," Bill added. "Kept it in good shape." A small shrug. "You wouldn't think."

The room held.

A week later, he said, "I didn't drink this weekend."

He didn't frame it as a decision.

"The weight of him was still there," he said. "Didn't feel like pushing it down."

He stopped there.

There was no attempt to make sense of it, no effort to draw a line between what had happened and what he was doing now. The thought of the man, the sense of himself in relation to him, and the absence of drinking remained alongside each other. Nothing in him moved to bring them together.

## Gabriella

Gabriella had always been able to find her way into a session. Even when something unsettled her, she could locate it quickly—name it, shape it, make it intelligible.

That day, she came in late.

"Sorry," she said, sitting down. She adjusted her sleeve, then stopped. "I knew what I wanted to say on the way here."

A brief pause.

"It made sense then."

She looked down, then back up.

"It doesn't now."

I didn't respond.

She sat with that, not rushing to replace it.

"I can feel where I would usually start," she said. "I'd tell you what happened this week. Or what I think it means." A faint shift in her expression. "That would settle it."

She paused again.

"I'm not doing that."

The room held.

"It's still there," she said. "Whatever it is." A quieter tone. "I just don't need to say it the way I usually do."

She didn't try again.

—

A few sessions later, she said, "I noticed something this week."

She took a breath but didn't continue immediately.

"I could feel myself starting to shut down," she said. "I knew exactly what I would normally do next."

She glanced at me briefly.

"I didn't do it."

Silence.

"I didn't try to push through it either." A slight shake of her head. "I just let it be there."

She sat back.

"It changed," she said after a moment. "Not because I figured it out."

She didn't elaborate.

—

Another time, she returned to a story she had told many times.

"I've said this before," she began. "About being in my room, waiting for my mom to come back."

She stopped.

"I know how I usually tell this."

A pause.

"It's different right now."

Her voice remained steady.

"I can feel how small I was."

Her hand moved slightly, then rested again.

"I'd normally explain that," she said. "Or tell you what it did to me." A faint exhale. "I don't need to."

Tears came, but she didn't move to shape them into anything further.

She remained with it, without adding to it.

What would once have been shaped into something she could say and understand no longer needed to arrive that way. The experience continued, altering without being secured.

## What It Asks of the Therapist

*Dynamic Flow* calls the therapist into participation in a rhythm rather than the guidance of a process. This is not a configuration of interpretation or insight delivery, but one of lived responsiveness within the analytic field. The therapist enters the movement of the patient's psyche—not to direct it, but to remain with it as it shifts, retracts, or unfolds in time. In this way, the therapist becomes a kind of internal rehearsal space: a partner in motion, participating in the movement rather than reflecting or stabilizing it from a fixed position.

This requires a tolerance for ambiguity. *Dynamic Flow* does not follow a linear arc or culminate in clear breakthroughs. It is patterned by subtle shifts—gaps in language, changes in tempo, tonal inflections that signal the psyche thinking aloud. The therapist's task is not to fix or translate these movements, but to allow space for them to continue. As Antonino Ferro writes, "The analyst must be ready to transform with the session," holding not a frame of certainty, but a willingness to be changed by what emerges.

With Gabriella, the countertransference may involve a pull toward coherence. Her intelligence and emotional precision can evoke admiration in the therapist—but also a subtle pressure to help her articulate or 'land' what she is circling. The therapist may feel compelled to affirm her insights too quickly, which risks interrupting her emerging capacity to stay with experience before it is named. There may also be an idealizing transferential echo—where the therapist feels moved by her process and must actively resist the wish to make it meaningful too soon. The task is to stay attuned without structuring, preserving the conditions in which flow, not conclusion, is possible.

With Bill, the countertransference may include a sense of under-engagement or a pressure to search for meaning that hasn't been articulated. His sparse narrative style and restrained emotional expression can create a felt uncertainty in the therapist—wondering whether therapeutic contact is occurring or whether it is being misread. At times, the therapist may feel overly invested in subtle shifts, interpreting them too strongly in an effort to 'catch' something real. The challenge is to tolerate the low-definition texture of the work and trust the slow unfolding of internal movement, even when it lacks clear markers.

Across both cases, the work is defined less by what the therapist does than by what is not done. The movement is sustained by the absence of intervention at the point where meaning would ordinarily be imposed. This requires more than restraint: the therapist relinquishes the need to know what the experience is becoming, or to bring it into a form that can be held and remains within the unfolding of the patient's experience without bringing it to rest.

## Justification for the Placement of this Configuration

*Dynamic Flow* follows *Revealing* and *Unconcealment,* where previously unformulated aspects of experience have entered psychic life but have not yet been stabilized or integrated within a coherent structure. What has emerged is present but not yet organized in a way that can be held in place. *Dynamic Flow* reflects the point at which the individual can remain with this material as it shifts, rather than converting it into meaning or withdrawing from it as it becomes less containable.

Its placement carries structural necessity within the movement of the process. It precedes *Repetition* and *A Nameless Dread,* where the psyche may be drawn back into unresolved configurations or brought into contact with forms of experience that exceed its existing capacity to contain them. Without *Dynamic Flow,* the movement from emergence into these later configurations would become more abrupt, increasing the likelihood of foreclosure or collapse. What becomes available here is a capacity to remain in motion without securing the experience—allowing what has come into view to continue without immediate resolution or defensive consolidation.

Clinically, this is not a stable achievement but a change in how experience is taken up. The individual begins to register the point at which meaning would ordinarily be imposed and does not follow that movement. Experience is neither avoided nor organized but allowed to proceed. In this sense, it differs from earlier defensive absences and from later states of disorganization. What appears here is not the return of content alone, but the emergence of a capacity to remain with it as it changes. In Winnicott's terms, this reflects a capacity to remain within experience without immediately organizing or resolving it, allowing something of it to unfold before it is taken up (Winnicott, 1971).

This is not surrender achieved, but the beginning of a sustained relation to experience in which closure is no longer required. What has been revealed does not settle into insight; it continues, altering without being brought to rest.

## Concluding Reflections

*Dynamic Flow* marks a shift in how experience is lived. What once required organization, explanation, or control is now allowed to continue without being brought to completion. The individual remains in contact with what is unfolding, without needing to secure it.

This does not produce clarity or resolution. It alters the relation to experience itself. Thought, feeling, and memory no longer have to be taken up in order to be held. They can register, shift, and persist without being shaped into meaning. What had been managed or foreclosed begins to move, not toward integration as an endpoint, but as an ongoing condition.

Gerald May (2004), writing in a spiritual context, describes a form of participation in which experience is not directed or resolved, but entered into. While his frame is theological, the structure he identifies—a relinquishing of control without withdrawal—finds a clinical parallel here. The individual does not step outside experience to understand it, nor collapse within it, but remains in contact as it changes.

In the therapeutic setting, this alters the nature of the work. The emphasis is no longer on arriving at insight, but on sustaining contact without imposing it. The therapist remains with the patient inside the movement of the material, without bringing it to rest. What develops is not a conclusion, but a capacity—the ability to remain with what is not yet formed and not require that it become so.

This is what prepares the ground for what follows. Not by resolving what has emerged, but by establishing that it can continue.

# 30 Repetition

*Repetition* marks a distinct configuration in the process of surrender, one that resists linear accounts of psychological change and simple developmental sequencing. Unlike compulsive reenactment, which returns to unrepresented trauma without transformation, this form of repetition carries the possibility of difference within the act of returning itself. It is not a defense against newness, but a re-encounter with earlier experience under altered internal and relational conditions.

Rather than signaling impasse or regression, repetition here reflects a change in how experience is borne. Psychic material re-emerges—not to be discharged or mastered, but to be held again. What once overwhelmed can now be encountered with greater symbolic capacity. The return is not identical; it is shaped by what has become available.

The Greek term *anamnesis*—to remember—points toward this process, though what occurs is not recollection alone. It is a re-encounter with experience that had not been fully taken up. As Bion (1962) describes, transformation depends on an oscillation between knowing and not knowing, in which each return alters what can be thought and felt.

Within the surrender process, *Repetition* becomes a way of remaining with what had previously been foreclosed, allowing return without the same compulsion toward discharge or avoidance. Its significance lies not in the fact of return, but in how it is sustained over time and within the analytic relation. What was once compelled can now be held without discharge or avoidance, remaining in contact with the self as it re-emerges. It is this change in psychic function that distinguishes *Repetition* here as a configuration within the surrender process.

## Jerome

Jerome had been in treatment long enough to know when he was avoiding something, but not long enough to stop himself from doing it. He arrived on time, as always, and sat with the studied calm of someone who knew how to survive silence.

"I almost cancelled today," he said after a while, eyes on the floor. "It felt pointless. Like I already knew what you'd say."

DOI: 10.4324/9781003795803-35

He let it sit there—not quite a complaint, not quite a challenge.

He exhaled. "You'd say I'm pushing too hard. That I'm doing the thing again—trying to get it right instead of..." He paused. "Staying with it."

Silence returned, not hostile but weighted. He shifted in his seat.

"It's not just you," he went on. "I feel it with everyone. Like they're holding up a scorecard I can't see. My team, my mother." A faint tightening in his jaw. "I hear it before anyone speaks—'you could've done better.'"

I said, "You're already inside the judgment before anything happens."

He looked up, meeting my gaze. "It's my mother's voice," he said. Then, after a beat, "No—it's not even that anymore. It's just...there."

He sat with that.

"I carry it," he added. "I set it up and then react to it. Like I hand people the script and then—" He stopped. A small shake of the head. "It just keeps going."

The words had come before. But not like this. There was less urgency in them now, less insistence that they land in a particular way.

"I keep saying I want to change," he said. "But when I get close to something that isn't already mapped out, I move. I explain it. I get ahead of it."

He paused.

"I can feel that happening right now."

He didn't continue.

The room held.

After a while, he said, more quietly, "Maybe it's not something I get out of."

A longer silence.

"I keep ending up here," he said. "But it doesn't feel exactly the same."

He frowned slightly, as if registering it rather than concluding it.

"It's like I'm not outside of it, trying to fix it." A pause. "I'm in it."

I stayed with him as he said it, without adding to it.

## Winston

He was on time for the first time in three weeks.

"I figured I'd make an appearance," he said, dropping his coat onto the chair instead of hanging it up like usual. He didn't look up.

I didn't comment on the timing.

"I had dinner with Olivia last weekend. I don't even know why I go. She orders for me like I'm incapable. Still has that habit of using my full name when she's mad." A half-laugh. "She was always better at rage than grief."

There was a rhythm to his speaking—quick, polished, just self-aware enough to pass for reflection. He had told versions of this before. The estranged sister, the same scenes returned to with slight variation.

"I'm not even angry anymore," he said. "It's just... efficient, I guess. I don't expect her to change. Or me."

He paused, briefly.

"But I still tell you about it."

The sentence remained between us.

He looked at me then—not searching, not asking—just long enough to register that I was there.

"I keep thinking maybe the story will land differently if I say it enough times," he said. "But it doesn't. It just—repeats."

I said, "And you hear it repeating."

He nodded, pressing his fingers into his temples.

"I always sound the same," he added. "Same tone, same ending. Like I already know where it goes before I start."

He let out a breath.

"I used to think I was broken in a way therapy couldn't touch. Like the best I could do was describe it well." A faint shift in his posture. "Keep it... contained."

The word lingered.

"I don't even know what I want from you most days," he said. "Just not silence. Not that feeling that nothing's happening."

I said, "Not just hearing it come back the same way."

Winston gave a small nod.

"Yeah." A pause. "Not just that."

Something slowed, almost imperceptibly.

"I don't know," he said. "It's like... even though it's the same thing, it's not exactly—" He stopped.

His gaze moved briefly toward me, then away.

"Not exactly nothing," he said.

I didn't add to it.

## What It Asks of the Therapist

The therapist must be able to recognize this shift without forcing it. The same words may be spoken, the same stories told, but their psychic position has altered. What had once been a closed circuit begins, subtly, to admit contact.

With Winston, this shift is difficult to locate. His repetitions arrive as polished narrative, edged with self-awareness but organized to prevent impact. The transference is flattened: I am positioned less as a distinct other than as a surface across which his speech can travel. The countertransference reflects this. There may be a pull toward disengagement, a sense of listening without being reached, or the temptation to intervene simply to interrupt the monotony. If I act from that pressure—by demanding novelty, redirecting, or sharpening interpretation—the repetition hardens back into defense. The work at this point is more exacting. I must remain within the repetition without collapsing into it, listening for where it thins—for the moment a phrase falters, or the narrative loses its grip. These are not dramatic shifts. They are easily overridden if I move too quickly.

With Jerome, repetition organizes more explicitly through transference. The expectation of evaluation enters the room before I speak. I am positioned as the one who will judge, confirm, or disappoint. His repetition is structured around anticipation—he performs, corrects, and pre-empts, attempting to manage how he will be received. The countertransference is correspondingly charged: a pressure to reassure, to meet him with precision, to avoid misstep. There may be a subtle wish to become the 'good' object he cannot locate. If I accept that position, even in softened form, the repetition continues unchanged. The task is not to oppose the pattern, but to refuse its completion—to remain present without confirming or correcting the anticipated outcome. In doing so, the repetition is no longer closed. It begins to be experienced rather than enacted.

*Repetition* requires the therapist to tolerate recurrence without converting it into meaning. The impulse to interpret, to differentiate, or to demonstrate progress may emerge as a defense against the strain of sameness within the analytic field. Here, interpretation can foreclose what is beginning to take shape. The therapist remains with the material as it recurs, allowing its internal variation to register before it is named, rather than organizing it prematurely into coherence.

What is asked, then, is not passivity but a precise form of restraint. The therapist must hold position within the repetition while relinquishing the need to alter its course. This involves a surrender of a particular kind: the surrender of efficacy as immediate action, the surrender of knowing in advance what constitutes change, and the surrender of the wish to bring the process to resolution.

Only under these conditions does *Repetition* begin to function differently. What returns is no longer identical. And it is within that slight difference—barely perceptible, easily lost—that the psyche begins to encounter itself in a new way.

## Justification for the Placement of this Configuration

Not all repetition belongs to surrender. In earlier configurations, repetition functions defensively—an attempt to manage psychic tension, avoid contact, or maintain cohesion where structure is fragile. What distinguishes *Repetition* is not the presence of return, but a change in its function. The material returns but is no longer sealed off from the self who encounters it. Something in the repetition reopens what had been foreclosed, allowing it to be met without discharge or mastery. It is not discharged, nor mastered, but held—again, and in relation.

*Repetition* emerges after *Dynamic Flow* and *Unconcealment*, once experience has begun to move without being immediately organized or resolved. Something has been contacted that was not previously available. But at this point, it cannot yet be sustained. The psyche returns to it—not to undo it, but because it cannot be held all at once.

What appears as repetition is this return.

It does not function as simple re-enactment. The material is not being discharged or avoided, nor is it being brought to completion. Instead, it reappears under altered internal conditions. What has been glimpsed begins to be encountered again, but now with a slightly expanded capacity to register it. The difference is not in the content, but in how it is borne.

Freud's (1915/2001) account of repetition as the return of the repressed remains foundational. What returns is not remembered as such but enacted—appearing without recognition and often outside narrative coherence. In *Repetition*, however, this return no longer functions primarily as resistance, but as a continuation of contact already established. It emerges after contact has begun to open and serves a different function within the analytic process. The psyche returns to what has been touched not to avoid it, but because it cannot yet be sustained in a continuous form. *Repetition* becomes the means by which this contact is gradually borne, without being forced into resolution or expelled from awareness.

For this reason, *Repetition* is not a delay in the process of surrender. It is the condition under which earlier contact can be stabilized without being fixed. The psyche does not move forward by leaving the material behind, but by returning to it until it can be borne without foreclosure or discharge. What develops is not a conclusion, but a capacity: the ability to remain in contact with what does not yet fully cohere.

This placement is necessary. Without this recursive engagement, the individual would either move prematurely toward resolution or retreat into defensive organization. *Repetition* allows the emerging material to be encountered repeatedly without being forced into meaning or expelled from awareness.

It is this capacity that prepares the transition to what follows, where symbolic organization begins to loosen and experience may no longer be held in the same way within the analytic field. *Repetition* marks the final point at which the psyche can still return, re-engage, and register difference within continuity, maintaining contact without the same degree of disorganization. What follows does not offer that return, and the movement of experience no longer permits the same form of re-engagement.

## Concluding Reflections

*Repetition* is easily mistaken for impasse. The same material returns, the same phrases reappear, and the movement of the work can seem to stall. But at this point in the process, something has shifted in how the return occurs. What repeats is no longer sealed off from contact. It returns under conditions in which it can be encountered, even if only partially.

What has not been integrated does not appear as narrative recall, but as recurrence—enacted, spoken, or lived without full recognition. Yet as the work deepens, this repetition begins to alter in function. The psyche returns not to discharge or avoid, but because it has come into contact with something it cannot yet sustain.

Bion's (1962) account of transformation helps to locate this shift. Experience is not taken in all at once, nor resolved through insight alone. It must be encountered repeatedly, in a rhythm of contact and loss, until it can be borne. Each return does not produce a conclusion, but a slight alteration in what can be registered. What was once overwhelming may begin to be held, if only momentarily, before it recedes again.

In *Repetition*, it is not something to be eliminated, but the condition under which contact stabilizes without becoming fixed or foreclosed. The patient does not move forward by leaving the material behind, but by returning to it without collapsing into it or moving prematurely to meaning, allowing continuity without resolution. The difference is often minimal—a hesitation, a shift in tone, a break in the continuity of the narrative—but it reflects a change in how the experience is carried within the analytic process.

This places a particular demand on the analytic situation. The work cannot be advanced by forcing differentiation or by naming what has not yet taken form. The *Repetition* must be allowed to proceed until its internal variation becomes perceptible. To interrupt it too soon is to restore its defensive function; to remain with it is to allow it to change.

*Repetition*, in this sense, marks the final point at which experience can still be returned to, re-engaged, and gradually borne within symbolic life.

What follows can no longer be rehearsed.

# Part V

# Releasement Level D

## At the Edge of Form

Temporary Attenuation and Dissolution of the Skin-Ego

*Releasement Level D* marks the furthest threshold in the process of surrender, where the organization of psychic life itself begins to loosen. Unlike prior configurations, which expand the psyche's *Capacity to Symbolize*, regulate, and metabolize experience, this level involves a loosening of psychic form as such. Crucially, this does not arise from psychic failure, but from psychic readiness within a sufficiently established structure. Only when prior functions—such as the *Capacity to Contain*, the *Capacity to Regress*, and *Subjective Appropriation*—have begun to consolidate can the self endure an encounter with experience at this level of unstructured intensity. This is not a breakdown, but a capacity: a rare psychic event made survivable by the stability that precedes it and continues to hold in its aftermath.

Didier Anzieu's concept of the skin-ego (1989) offers a frame for understanding what gives way here. The skin-ego functions as a protective psychic envelope, modeled on the infant's experience of the body's skin as a boundary for sensation and selfhood. In ordinary functioning, it organizes perception and regulates affect. At this final level of surrender, that envelope does not rupture in a traumatic sense, but becomes temporarily altered. At times, it is attenuated—its boundary functions softened enough to allow contact with previously unformulated material. At others, it may approach a temporary dissolution: a momentary loss of psychic enclosure in which symbolic mediation gives way and raw affect dominates the field. These are not identical experiences, but variations in how the psyche comes into contact with what exceeds its usual form. Both register a proximity to psychic limits, and to the possibility of reconstitution.

What is encountered is not a collapse of ego functions, but a shift in the skin-ego's protective capacities. The envelope thins, not because it has failed, but because the psyche has become able—under specific conditions—to tolerate what lies beyond it. What would previously have

DOI: 10.4324/9781003795803-36

overwhelmed can now be approached without immediate foreclosure. This paradox—that only a sufficiently established structure can permit its own loosening—defines this releasement level.

Bion's concept of nameless dread (1962) captures this exposure: the emergence of emotional experience that has not undergone alpha-function and therefore cannot yet be thought. In such moments, symbolic function recedes. Insight is not available. What becomes essential is reverie—the analyst's capacity to receive, hold, and metabolize what the patient cannot yet experience as their own. Reverie here is not interpretive but containing. It allows the patient to borrow a form of psychic organization until something of the experience can begin to be reintroduced into symbolic life. While Bion situates such states in relation to failures of containment, this model locates them, at this level, as arising not from deficit but from a capacity that has been sufficiently established to permit contact with what would otherwise be unendurable.

Neurobiological accounts of affect regulation describe a corresponding shift at the level of brain function. Under conditions of overwhelming affect, regulatory and integrative functions associated with the prefrontal cortex diminish, while subcortical systems become more dominant. The result is not simply heightened emotion, but a reduction in the capacity to organize experience into narrative or thought. These shifts echo what psychoanalysis describes as a temporary loss of symbolic mediation, underscoring that what is encountered here is not only a subjective experience, but a change in the conditions under which experience can be organized at all.

This level of surrender cannot be summoned. It arises only under conditions of sufficient psychic safety, and even then, only intermittently. It is not integration, but exposure. And yet, this exposure is only possible because structure has already been established. The psyche can approach formlessness because it retains, however faintly, the capacity to return from it.

# 31 A Nameless Dread

This level of surrender marks a furthest threshold—one that departs from the forms of integration seen in prior configurations and moves toward direct psychic exposure. *A Nameless Dread* arrives as an unmediated encounter: an intrusion of something too raw to symbolize, too immediate to be held within existing structures of meaning. Paradoxically, such an encounter becomes possible only where internal capacities have been sufficiently established and can continue to hold in its presence. What might once have shattered the self can now, under rare conditions, be endured without immediate disintegration.

This is not the psychic flooding of panic, which still presumes a self who feels overwhelmed. *A Nameless Dread* arises when that very organization is suspended—when what is felt cannot yet be known, owned, or located. It is not simply disorganization; it precedes organization. What shifts is not resolution, but the psyche's capacity to remain in contact with what cannot yet be made into experience.

Until this point, even the deeper capacities cultivated through surrender—containment, regression, symbolic appropriation—have unfolded within structure. Here, something more primitive emerges: not what has been repressed, but what has never been fully available to thought. The psyche comes into contact with what it could not previously register. These encounters are often brief, partial, or somatically marked. They do not culminate in resolution. They recur, each time altering what can be encountered and endured.

If earlier levels of surrender were organized through the development of psychic structure, this involves a loosening of that organization under conditions in which it can still be maintained. Rhythm no longer functions in the same way. Containment does not disappear but becomes less structuring, less determinative of how experience is held. Experience is encountered with reduced mediation, without being entirely unheld.

Bion's concept of nameless dread (1962) captures this exposure: the emergence of unprocessed emotional experience that has not undergone alpha-function and therefore cannot yet be thought. In such moments, raw sensory-affective elements dominate the field. There is no distance from experience, and no capacity to transform it into meaning.

DOI: 10.4324/9781003795803-37

Bion described such states in relation to failures of early containment. Here, the same psychic substance is encountered under different conditions. It does not signal collapse, but a capacity to approach what would otherwise remain foreclosed. What changes is not the material itself, but the conditions under which it can be borne.

In analytic work, such moments cannot be met with interpretation. They require the analyst's capacity for reverie: to receive, hold, and metabolize what the patient cannot yet experience as their own. This is not an intervention in the usual sense, but a form of presence that maintains contact without imposing structure.

Melanie Klein (1946) located similar states in the earliest phases of psychic life, where anxiety takes the form of potential annihilation and the self lacks the cohesion to contain its own experience. Here, such conditions may be revisited—not as regression alone, but as contact with levels of experience that were never fully integrated.

Mystical traditions describe a comparable terrain. Dionysius the Areopagite referred to it as *apohaeresis*: not illumination, but stripping—a radical un-forming in which one is divested of what can be known or grasped. In this sense, *Nameless Dread* is not only a clinical phenomenon, but a form of contact with what lies beyond representation.

This is not an achievement. It cannot be produced or sustained at will. It arises intermittently, and often at the limits of what can be endured. But when it occurs in the presence of another who does not turn away, it becomes survivable.

## Winston

He had been talking about something familiar—someone from his residency years, a patient who used to fake symptoms for pills. He smiled as he spoke, in that way he sometimes did, as though watching himself from across the room.

Then he went quiet.

At first, it felt like a pause. Then something gave. His shoulders rounded. His eyes no longer tracked.

After a moment, he said, "I think I was gone just now."

I stayed where I was.

"I don't mean gone like spaced out," he said, already sounding uncertain. "It was like I was there, but I didn't know who was here." His fingers pressed into the armrest, not gripping, but testing. "Everything felt thin. Like the room was... too big."

I said, "You were here, but not held together."

He looked at me briefly, then away. "Yeah... but not falling apart either." A pause. "That's the part I don't get."

He wasn't withdrawing. There was no dulling, no retreat. Something had come forward without form, and it was arriving faster than he could take it in.

"It wasn't a memory," he said. "I didn't see anything." He swallowed. "It was like... there was no 'me' to see it. I just felt like I was being looked at from the inside."

I didn't move to meet that with meaning.

The room shifted. Not empty—more dense. As though something had entered without shape, without edges. It did not organize into feeling, or thought, or image. It pressed.

He did not look at me. I did not reach for him.

"There's something here," I said, not to define it, but to keep it from disappearing.

He nodded faintly.

We sat inside it—without language, without direction. Not absence, but something prior to it. The dread between us, not his and not mine, but present enough to be shared.

Later, weeks later, he said, "I think that was the first time I wasn't trying to be anyone. Not even with you." He paused. "I didn't know what you saw... and that scared me." Another pause. "But I didn't leave."

## Jerome

Jerome had always come prepared. Articulate, driven, hyper-attuned to nuance. He thought analytically about everything—his relationships, his dreams, his childhood. For years, he had stayed ahead of his pain by naming it before it could reach him.

One afternoon, several years into the work, he began the session in silence. His body was tense, as if holding something in place.

I waited.

When he finally spoke, it wasn't in his usual tone. It was flat, almost childlike.

"I can't... think."

"What's happening right now?" I asked.

"I mean... I don't know what I'm feeling." He shook his head slightly. "I know I should. I know I'm supposed to say something, but all I know is that I feel sick and my chest won't open."

"It might not be something to understand yet."

He swallowed hard. "I don't want to cry. It's not that I'm trying not to. It just won't come." A pause. "But I'm full. Like—like I'm drowning in something with no name."

The words trailed off. He didn't look at me.

"I think I've been scared for so long, I stopped knowing what scared feels like."

I didn't move to organize it.

His hands were folded tightly in his lap, not in control, but bracing. His gaze fixed just to the side of me. The words were no longer working for him. They didn't reach far enough.

"There's something here," I said, not to name it, but to keep it from slipping back into structure.

He nodded once, almost imperceptibly.

We stayed with it. Not something hidden, but something not yet able to take form. It did not gather into feeling or thought. It pressed from underneath, without direction.

Later, he said he didn't remember much from that session. Not absence—more that it hadn't taken shape. "Something shifted," he said. "Not like a breakthrough." He paused. "More like something gave way."

What followed wasn't clarity. Language came slowly. Images arrived without context. There was a dream he could not recount without his body tightening. There were moments he described standing next to his own fear, unable to approach it or step away.

He didn't ask what it meant.

He didn't want it translated.

He wanted to stay in the room.

## What It Asks of the Therapist

At this threshold, the therapist is asked not to intervene but to remain—to sustain a presence at the limits of what the psyche can tolerate. These are not moments for meaning, but for a form of containment that does not yet organize what it holds. Interpretation, here, would not deepen the work, but displace it—imposing structure where none has yet taken shape.

The dread encountered at this level is not fear in the usual sense, but a psychic event preceding the conditions for thought. What the patient encounters cannot yet be represented. It arrives as intensity without image, without narrative, without differentiation. And yet, this exposure is only possible because something in the psyche has already developed the capacity to survive it. The patient does not enter this state empty-handed; they arrive with a history of having been held—within the analytic relationship and, at least in part, within themselves. What is absent is not structure entirely, but the ability to use it in the moment.

The therapist, in turn, must tolerate the pressure to act without yielding to it. This is not neutrality, but a sustained internal effort not to organize what has not yet formed. One listens not for meaning, but for shifts in the field—for the emergence of something that does not yet know itself. In the transference, the patient does not present an experience so much as expose the analyst to it. The countertransference often carries this directly: a pull toward confusion, toward urgency, toward premature coherence, or toward a kind of inward thinning. The task is not to resolve these pressures, but to register them without converting them into intervention.

It becomes essential to differentiate between forms of psychic absence. Not all silence is the same. "I can't think" may signal withdrawal, or it may indicate contact with something that has not yet entered thought. The distinction is not made through content, but through the quality of the moment—its density, its direction, its insistence. In some instances, the mind has turned away; in others, it is being approached by something it cannot yet receive.

With Jerome, the dread emerged within a psyche organized around mastery. His reliance on language had long kept certain affects at a distance. What appeared in the analytic field was not the arrival of new material, but the failure of his usual means of containing it. The transference carried an expectation—subtle but present—that the analyst would help him recover coherence. The countertransference registered the pull to do exactly that: to name, to clarify, to restore continuity. To follow that pull would have re-established the defense. The work required remaining with him as that coherence faltered, without stepping in to rebuild it. His dread did not come from an absence of structure, but from its suspension.

With Winston, the field was different. The dread did not follow the breakdown of an established structure but emerged where structure had never fully formed. The transference did not seek restoration so much as proximity—an exposure without clear expectation. The countertransference was correspondingly more somatic, at times carrying a sense of drift, or a pull toward disengagement. The risk was not premature interpretation, but subtle withdrawal. What was required was a steadiness that did not organize the experience but did not leave it unheld. The work was less about allowing something to fall apart, and more about not turning away from something that had never cohered.

In both instances, the analyst is drawn toward action—toward restoring, naming, stabilizing. The discipline lies in not taking up that role too soon. The patient is not without support in these moments; the support is the analyst's capacity to remain in contact without altering the state.

These moments are rarely retained as narrative. They are not remembered as events but appear later as shifts—less urgency to defend, greater tolerance for states that previously required evacuation, a different relation to not knowing. Something has been endured without being transformed, and that endurance alters what becomes possible thereafter.

## Justification for the Placement of this Configuration

The placement of *A Nameless Dread* at the furthest reach of the surrender model reflects its position as a limit condition rather than a culmination. It does not complete the process but brings it to a point at which what emerges can no longer be carried further through ordinary psychic means. What emerges here does not build on prior configurations in a linear sense; it tests the extent to which those configurations sustain contact with what the psyche cannot yet organize.

This threshold does not arise from deficit but from capacity. Only where the psyche has developed the ability to contain, to remain in contact with uncertainty, and to allow experience to unfold without immediate structuring can it approach this level. Earlier configurations establish the conditions under which something unformulated can be encountered without immediate evacuation, allowing contact without premature reorganization. Without that groundwork, such exposure would not be endured—it would be foreclosed or converted into more familiar forms of distress.

The movement of the model does not proceed toward greater clarity, but toward an increased tolerance for what resists clarity. Each configuration extends the range of what can be experienced without premature resolution, widening the field of what can be held without transformation. At this level, that movement reaches its limit. The psyche no longer works to transform experience into meaning, but to remain in contact with what cannot yet be made meaningful, where experience persists without symbolic resolution. This is not a failure of the process, but its furthest expression.

This dread has been described as a kind of primitive resistance to change—not in the sense of defensive avoidance, but as a response to the loss of familiar structures of experience. What is feared is not simply what will come, but the dissolution of what has organized the self up to that point. In this way, the dread signals proximity to transformation, not its absence.

The inclusion of mystical literature serves to articulate this terrain more precisely. These traditions have long attempted to describe inner conditions that exceed representation—states in which familiar structures of meaning fall away without immediate replacement. Their language, while shaped by theological concerns, often attends closely to the experience of disorientation, exposure, and the suspension of knowing.

Accounts of what has been described as a 'dark night' capture this shift with particular clarity. What is lost is not simply comfort or coherence, but the very means by which experience has previously been known. The individual does not encounter new meaning, but the absence of the forms that once made meaning possible. What remains is not emptiness, but an encounter with something that cannot yet be taken up into thought.

In this context, nameless dread is not understood as breakdown, but as contact with what lies beyond the current reach of symbolization. It appears only when prior structures can be suspended without immediate collapse. For this reason, it cannot be placed earlier in the model without distorting its function. To encounter this level without sufficient development would not result in exposure, but in fragmentation or defensive retreat.

Placed at the furthest reach of the model, this clarifies that surrender does not culminate in integration, insight, or resolution. It extends toward the capacity to remain in contact with what exceeds those forms. The psyche does not resolve the experience; it endures it. And in that endurance—however brief, however incomplete—the range of what can be lived without evacuation is altered.

This is the outer limit of the model: not a final state to be achieved, but the furthest point at which the psyche can remain present to itself without turning away.

## Concluding Reflections

*A Nameless Dread* does not confront the subject with trauma alone, but with the limits of psychic form—the point at which meaning gives way and something remains that cannot yet be taken up into thought. What appears is not fear of something, but fear without object: an intensity that does not organize, does not resolve, and cannot be made to cohere through effort. To remain in contact with such a state requires what has been described as negative capability—a capacity to tolerate not knowing without moving prematurely to restore coherence. What emerges in these moments cannot yet be thought. It must first be endured.

This places a particular demand on the analytic relationship. The work is no longer to uncover or to interpret, but to remain in contact with what resists both. The analyst is drawn toward action—toward naming, stabilizing, restoring—but to do so too quickly would be to displace the experience itself. What is required instead is a steadiness that does not organize what has not yet formed and does not withdraw in the face of what cannot be metabolized. The patient does not borrow meaning here, but the capacity to stay.

This threshold is not encountered once, nor is it sustained. It appears, recedes, and returns under different conditions, each time altering what can be borne without retreat. It does not resolve. It changes the relation to what does not resolve.

To refuse this level of experience is not simply to avoid distress. It is to remain organized around what can already be known, already managed, already survived. Life narrows accordingly. Experience becomes shaped in advance—anticipated, contained, rendered familiar before it has the chance to arrive. What is lost is not intensity, but range: the capacity to be affected by what exceeds expectation, to encounter what cannot be predicted or controlled.

At its furthest reach, surrender exposes the psyche to what it cannot master. This is not a collapse into meaninglessness, but a contact with something prior to meaning—a condition in which the self is no longer secured by its own structures. There is risk here. Without sufficient development, such exposure would fragment rather than deepen. But when it can be endured, even briefly, something shifts. Not resolution, not clarity, but an expansion in what can be lived without immediate transformation.

In this sense, the cost of not surrendering is not failure, but constriction. The structures that protect the self remain intact, but they also limit what can be encountered. The psyche is preserved, but at the expense of its reach.

The surrender model traces the conditions under which this reach becomes possible. It does not lead to a final state, but to an altered relation to experience itself—one in which the individual can remain in contact with what does not yet have form, without turning away. And in that contact, something of aliveness returns—not as resolution, but as the capacity to remain where one would otherwise have withdrawn.

# 32 Reflections on the Structure of Surrender

The concept of surrender has long circulated within both psychoanalytic and philosophical discourse, yet it has often done so without precise differentiation. At times it has been conflated with submission, resignation, or collapse; at other times it has appeared in spiritual literature as a transformative experience that seems difficult to translate into psychological language.

The model presented in this book attempts to clarify this terrain by identifying a series of experiential conditions through which surrender becomes psychologically possible. Rather than describing a sequence of achievements or a fixed developmental path, the model offers a conceptual framework for recognizing recurring configurations of experience that may emerge within psychoanalytic work when defensive organization begins to loosen.

From this perspective, the configurations described throughout the book are not intended as prescriptive steps but as observations of how psychic life reorganizes under particular relational and psychological conditions. They reflect movements within experience that become visible in the analytic field as patients encounter aspects of themselves that had previously remained outside awareness, coming into contact with what had not yet been taken up within psychic life.

Seen in this way, the model functions less as a ladder of development than as a kind of psychoanalytic field map—an attempt to name the shifting experiential conditions through which surrender becomes possible within analytic work.

## The Structure of the Surrender Model

The model described in this book is not intended to function as a sequence of psychological achievements or as a prescriptive path through treatment. Rather, it offers a conceptual map of experiential conditions that may arise within analytic work as defensive organization loosens. These conditions appear in different ways across analytic processes, sometimes gradually and sometimes unexpectedly, as aspects of psychic life that had previously remained outside awareness come into contact with the analytic field.

DOI: 10.4324/9781003795803-38

For this reason, the model may be understood less as a linear progression than as a field of related psychological movements. Each configuration names a particular organization of experience that may become observable in analytic work under specific relational and internal conditions. Some of these configurations establish foundational capacities associated with deeper psychic contact, while others reflect more destabilizing encounters with previously unformulated aspects of experience as they come into view. Although the configurations are presented sequentially for clarity, clinical observation suggests that patients may move among them in complex and nonlinear ways, returning to earlier experiential conditions under altered internal organization.

Within the model are foundational capacities that make surrender psychologically conceivable. In the *Closed* position, defensive organization is dominant, and surrender is experienced primarily as threat. The *Capacity to Depend* introduces the possibility of relying upon another mind within the analytic relationship. *Open-Ended Attention* allows the patient to remain in contact with experience without immediately organizing or defending against it, while the *Capacity to Regress* permits a temporary loosening of adult defensive structures so that earlier emotional states may emerge within the safety of the analytic setting.

These conditions are often present in relation to what the model describes as *Releasement*, a process in which the patient relinquishes defensive control over psychic experience. In its earlier movements, the psyche develops capacities associated with tolerating previously defended emotional states, including *Tolerance of Frustration, Readiness for Anxiety*, the *Capacity to Symbolize*, and *Subjective Appropriation*. At times, the relinquishment of volitional control may occur through experiential states such as *Non-Willing, Contemplation, Ecstasy*, and *Doubt*—moments in which the individual encounters psychic life with less reliance on deliberate control or defensive organization.

At times, the loosening of defensive organization may be accompanied by a more sustained reorganization of psychic life. Within this phase, several transformational movements may emerge. The *Shift* represents a change in the individual's relationship to their own psychic life, often accompanied by a growing sense of gratitude, humility, or altered perception of experience. In *Revealing* and *Unconcealment*, aspects of the self that had previously been hidden or defended against begin to come into view. *Dynamic Flow* reflects an increased flexibility within psychic functioning, allowing the individual to move more freely between internal states without rigid defensive interference.

Within this field of experience, conditions may arise in which experience becomes more available to the self. *Wisdom* reflects a form of experiential understanding that emerges from lived encounter rather than abstract reasoning. *Love*, in this context, represents an openness toward the self and others that becomes possible when defensive structures no longer dominate relational life.

The model also recognizes that analytic work rarely proceeds in a straight line. *Repetition* acknowledges that individuals return to earlier experiential conditions multiple times, encountering them under altered internal organization rather than simply repeating what has already occurred. What may appear as repetition can instead reflect a deepening of psychic contact with previously defended material as it re-emerges under different conditions of contact.

At its furthest threshold, the surrender process may involve contact with what Bion described as *Nameless Dread,* a limit condition of psychic experience. This refers to an encounter with unformulated emotional experience that precedes symbolization. Within the context of analytic work, such moments may become survivable under conditions in which the psyche can sustain contact without immediate collapse.

Viewed together, these configurations do not describe a fixed developmental ladder but rather a field of experiential possibilities that may become visible in analytic work as defensive organization softens. The model is therefore offered not as a prescription for treatment but as a shared vocabulary through which clinicians, teachers, and students may recognize and discuss the subtle movements of surrender as they emerge within analytic practice.

## The Lifelong Nature of Surrender

What becomes evident through clinical observation is that surrender does not occur once and for all. Rather, it represents an ongoing movement within psychic life. Individuals may revisit earlier forms of experience many times over the course of treatment and throughout their lives, encountering them under different internal conditions.

This cyclical quality reflects the dynamic nature of the psyche itself. Psychic organization is continually reworked as new experiences arise and previously defended material comes into thought and feeling under altered conditions of contact. The configurations described in this model do not represent final destinations but recurring movements within psychic life, returning in different forms as internal organization shifts.

Understanding these movements makes it possible to differentiate experiences that might otherwise appear similar while reflecting very different psychic conditions. In this sense, the model serves less as a map of therapeutic progress than as a conceptual framework for recognizing the varied ways the psyche comes into contact with itself.

## Final Reflections

The model of surrender described in this book does not present a sequence of psychological achievements but identifies experiential configurations that may emerge as defensive organization loosens. These states may appear in different ways across analytic work—sometimes gradually and sometimes unexpectedly—as aspects of psychic life that had previously remained inaccessible come into contact with the analytic field.

Seen in this light, surrender is not a therapeutic goal to be pursued but a phenomenon that becomes visible under particular internal conditions. The analyst does not produce these moments through technique alone; rather, they arise within the analytic relationship under conditions in which previously defended experience comes into contact with thought and feeling, without immediate reorganization. The configurations within the surrender model reflect different ways in which that contact may occur and be sustained within the analytic field.

For clinicians, the usefulness of the model lies in its capacity to help differentiate experiences that might otherwise appear similar while reflecting very different psychic conditions. Moments of openness may signal regression, releasement, symbolic emergence, or encounters with unformulated affect. Recognizing these distinctions deepens clinical understanding and supports the analyst's capacity to remain with what is unfolding in the analytic field.

For teachers and students of psychoanalysis, the model offers a framework for discussing phenomena that are frequently encountered in training but not always named with precision. By articulating these experiential patterns, the aim is to make possible clearer dialogue about the subtle movements of psychic life that occur within analytic work.

The surrender model is therefore best understood as a working vocabulary—an attempt to give language to experiences that remain complex, evolving, and open to further elaboration within the psychoanalytic community.

# Appendix: Methodology and Expansion of the Surrender Model

## Introduction to the Model's Origins

The surrender model presented in this book originated in the author's doctoral research, first developed in a dissertation published in 2008. The original project sought to examine how experiences described as surrender appear across psychological and contemplative literature and to organize these phenomenological descriptions of experience into a preliminary conceptual framework.

Through this work, recurring experiential patterns became discernible across texts and early clinical observations. These patterns formed the basis for the initial formulation of the surrender model, which was first introduced in that study and is further developed in the present volume.

While surrender is often described in philosophical and mystical traditions as an individual transformation, early clinical observation suggested that in psychoanalytic work such experiences frequently arise within the relational field between patient and analyst. This observation became a central organizing question for the development of the model.

In its earliest psychoanalytic formulation, the model was conceived as a way of mapping recurring experiential configurations that appear within analytic work as defensive organization loosens. The structure was initially explored in relation to Bion's analytic grid (1963) as a means of conceptualizing how different forms of experience come into contact with thought, symbolization, and emotional life within the analytic field.

The present book expands that initial framework by situating the model more fully within contemporary psychoanalytic theory and by examining how these experiential configurations appear in clinical practice.

## Textual and Theoretical Analysis

The initial development of the surrender model involved the thematic analysis of psychological and contemplative texts using the approach described by Boyatzis (1998). The aim of this analysis was to identify recurring phenomenological descriptions of experiential conditions associated with surrender, including relinquishment of control, openness to experience, and encounters with aspects of psychic life that exceed ordinary ego organization.

Analysis proceeded through a hybrid coding process incorporating three complementary approaches:

**Inductive coding.** Conceptual categories were identified within the material.

**Prior-research-driven coding.** Existing models of therapeutic change, particularly those proposed by Gendlin, Greenberg, and Safran, informed the interpretation of these themes.

**Theory-driven coding.** Psychoanalytic concepts concerning transformation, regression, and symbolization provided an additional framework for organizing these observations.

Through this iterative process, recurring experiential patterns were identified and articulated in the preliminary structure that later became the surrender model.

## Psychoanalytic Conceptualization

Subsequent work sought to situate these observations more explicitly within psychoanalytic theory. Contributions from Bion, Winnicott, André Green, Didier Anzieu, Roussillon, and other psychoanalytic thinkers provided conceptual language for understanding how defensive organization loosens, and how previously unformulated emotional experience comes into contact with symbolization within analytic work.

Within this framework, surrender came to be understood not simply as an internal psychological state but as a phenomenon that becomes observable within the analytic relationship under particular relational conditions.

## Application to Clinical Material

The model was further developed through reflection on clinical material drawn from the author's analytic practice. Observations of analytic encounters led to a reconsideration of the provisional configurations identified in earlier work in relation to the unfolding of clinical process.

Clinical material clarified how surrender-related experiences appear within treatment through shifts in tone, silence, symbolic expression, and emotional contact. These observations also demonstrated the nonlinear nature of the process, as patients frequently revisit earlier experiential conditions under different internal conditions.

## The Role of the Analyst

Clinical observation also suggested that surrender is not experienced solely by the patient but may involve shifts within the analytic field itself. Moments in which patients relinquish defensive control can evoke corresponding states of receptivity or openness in the analyst.

At the same time, such moments may also challenge the analyst. Intensified transference dynamics can evoke pressures toward certainty, control, or premature interpretation. In this sense, the analyst may also encounter the need to relinquish certain forms of technical or psychological control in order to remain receptive to experience within the analytic field.

Surrender within analytic work therefore does not occur on one side of the relationship alone but may involve a corresponding loosening of defensive organization within both participants.

## The Integration of Mystical and Psychoanalytic Perspectives

Although the present work approaches surrender primarily through psychoanalytic theory, earlier engagement with mystical literature continues to inform the model's attention to lived experience. Mystical writings often provide phenomenological descriptions of states of relinquishment, openness, and transformation with a precision that conveys experiential qualities that may be difficult to articulate in psychological language.

Rather than merging mystical and psychoanalytic frameworks, the present work treats these traditions as distinct yet complementary sources of insight. Mystical literature offered descriptive accounts of experiential states, while psychoanalysis provides a relational and clinical framework for understanding how similar experiences appear within analytic practice.

## Implications for Future Inquiry

The surrender model described in this book is offered as a provisional conceptual framework rather than a closed theoretical system. Further inquiry may explore how surrender-related phenomena appear across different psychoanalytic traditions, cultural contexts, and therapeutic settings.

In articulating a vocabulary for recognizing these phenomenological configurations of experience, the model supports continued dialogue about movements of psychic transformation within the psychoanalytic community.

# References


Almaas, A. H. (2002). *Spacecruiser inquiry: True guidance for the inner journey.* Shambhala.

Anzieu, D. (1989). *The skin ego* (C. Turner, Trans.). Karnac Books.

Avery, P., & Heath-Stubbs, J. (Eds.). (2003). *The Penguin book of Arabic verse.* Penguin Classics.

Benjamin, J. (2018). *Beyond doer and done to: Recognition theory, intersubjectivity and the third.* Routledge.

Bick, E. (1968) The experience of the skin in early object-relations. *International Journal of Psycho-Analysis* 49, 484–486.

Bion, W. R. (1962). Learning from experience. In C. Mawson (Ed.) (2014), *The complete works of W. R. Bion, volume IV: 1940–1962* (pp. 261–365). Karnac.

Bion, W. R. (1963). Elements of psycho-analysis. In C. Mawson (Ed.) (2014), *The complete works of W. R. Bion, volume V: 1963–1965* (pp. 1–86). Karnac.

Bion, W. R. (1967). Memory and desire. In C. Mawson (Ed.) (2014), *The complete works of W.R. Bion, volume VI: 1965–1970* (pp. 7–17). Karnac.

Bion, W. R. (1970). Attention and interpretation. In C. Mawson (Ed.) (2014), *The complete works of W. R. Bion, volume VI: 1965–1970* (pp. 211–330). Karnac.

Bion, W. R. (1971). The grid. In C. Mawson (Ed.) (2014), *The complete works of W. R. Bion, volume X: 1971–1977* (pp. 6–32). Karnac.

Bollas, C. (1981). Treatment of primitive mental states. *International Journal of Psycho-Analysis,* 62, 251–255.

Bollas, C. (1987). *The shadow of the object: Psychoanalysis of the unthought known.* Columbia University Press.

Bowlby, J. (1969). *Attachment and loss: Vol. 1. Attachment.* Basic Books.

Bowlby, J. (1973). *Attachment and loss: Vol. 2. Separation: Anxiety and anger.* Basic Books.

Caputo, J. D. (1978). *The mystical element in Heidegger's thought.* Ohio University Press.

Coltart, N. (1985). Slouching towards Bethlehem... or thinking the unthinkable in psychoanalysis. *International Review of Psycho-Analysis,* 12, 3–14.

Dante Alighieri. (c.1308–1314) *Inferno.* Translated by Allen Mandelbaum. Bantam Books, 1982.

Ferro, A. (2005). *Seeds of illness, seeds of recovery: The genesis of suffering and the role of psychoanalysis.* Routledge.

Ferro, A. (2006). *Psychoanalysis as therapy and storytelling.* Routledge.

Ferro, A. (2017). *Psychoanalysis and narration: Way beyond interpretation*. Routledge.

Fonagy, P., Gergely, G., Jurist, E. L., & Target, M. (2002). *Affect regulation, mentalization, and the development of the self*. Other Press.

Freud, S. (1911). Formulations on the two principles of mental functioning. In J. Strachey (Ed. & Trans.), *The standard edition of the complete psychological works of Sigmund Freud* (Vol. 12, 213–226). Vintage.

Freud, S. (1912). The dynamics of transference. In J. Strachey (Ed. & Trans.), *The standard edition of the complete psychological works of Sigmund Freud* (Vol. 12, 97–108). Vintage.

Freud, S. (1915/2001). Repression. In J. Strachey (Ed. & Trans.), *The standard edition of the complete psychological works of Sigmund Freud* (Vol. 14, 141–158). Vintage.

Freud, S., & Breuer, J. (2001). Studies on hysteria. In J. Strachey, Ed. & Trans.), *The standard edition of the complete psychological works of Sigmund Freud* (Vol. 2). Vintage.

Gendlin, E. T. (1981). *Focusing*. Bantam Books.

Gendlin, E. T. (1997). *Experiencing and the creation of meaning: A philosophical and psychological approach to the subjective*. Northwestern University Press.

Ghent, E. (1990). Masochism, submission, surrender: Masochism as a perversion of surrender. *Contemporary Psychoanalysis*, 26 (1), 108–136.

Green, A. (1983/1993). The dead mother. In *Narcissisme de vie, narcissisme de mort* [Originally published 1983; translated by Erika Kittler]. *Psyche*, 47 (3), 205–240.

Green, A. (1999). *The work of the negative* (A. Weller, Trans.). Free Association Books.

Greenberg, L., & Safran, J. (1987). *Emotion in psychotherapy*. Guilford Press.

Hafiz. (2010). *Faces of love* (D. Davis, Trans.). Mage Publishers.

Heidegger, M. (1927). *Being and time* (J. Macquarrie & E. Robinson, Trans.) (1962). Harper & Row.

James, W. (1890). *The principles of psychology* (Vol. 1) (1950) New York: Dover.

Keats, J. (1817). Letter to George and Tom Keats, December 1817, in *Selected letters of John Keats* (ed. Robert Gittings, 1970). Oxford University Press.

Klein, M. (1946). Notes on some schizoid mechanisms. In *Envy and gratitude and other works 1946–1963*. Vintage.

Klein, M. (1957). *Envy and gratitude and other works 1946–1963*. (1975). Hogarth Press and the Institute of Psycho-Analysis.

Kris, E. (1952). *Psychoanalytic explorations in art*. New York: International Universities Press.

Lewis, F. (2000). *Rumi: Past and present, East and West*. Oneworld Publications.

Luibhéid, C. (1987). *Pseudo-Dionysius: The complete works* (C. Luibhéid, Trans.; P. Rorem, Ed.). Mahwah, NJ: Paulist Press.

May, G. G. (2004). *The dark night of the soul: A psychiatrist explores the connection between darkness and spiritual growth* (T. B. Kirsch, Ed.). HarperOne. (Original work unpublished).

McGuire, W. (Ed.). (1974). *The Freud/Jung letters: The correspondence between Sigmund Freud and C.G. Jung*. Princeton University Press.

Moore, T. (2004). *Dark nights of the soul: A guide to finding your way through life's ordeals*. Gotham Books/Penguin Group.

Ogden, T. H. (1994). The analytic third: Working with intersubjective clinical facts. *The International Journal of Psychoanalysis*, 75 (1), 3–19.

Ogden, T. H. (1983). The concept of internal object relations. *International Journal of Psychoanalysis*, 64, 227–241.

Ogden, T. H. (2005). *Subjects of analysis*. Jason Aronson.

Rickard, K. M. (2008). *An exploration of the process of opening to experiencing mystical knowledge* (Publication No. 3338432) [Doctoral dissertation, California Institute of Integral Studies]. ProQuest Dissertations Publishing.

Rossi, V. (1995). Perennial philosophy and the recovery of a theological vision. *Journal of the Fellowship of St. Alban and St. Sergius*, 28, 35–47.

Roussillon, R. (2010). Working through and its various models. *International Journal of Psychoanalysis*, 91 (6), 1405–1417.

Roussillon, R. (2011). *Primitive agony and symbolization*. Routledge.

Segal, H. (1957). Notes on symbol formation. *International Journal of Psychoanalysis*, 38, 391–397.

Spillius, E. B., Milton, J., Garvey, P., Couve, C., & Steiner, D. (Eds.). (2011). *The new dictionary of Kleinian thought*. Routledge.

St. John of the Cross. (c.1577–1579). *Dark night of the soul* (E. Allison Peers, Trans.). (1959). Image Books.

St. John of the Cross. (c.1577–1579). *Dark night of the soul* (M. Starr, Trans.). (2002). Riverhead Books.

Underhill, E. (1993). *Mysticism: A study in the nature and development of spiritual consciousness*. Oneworld.

Weil, S. (2009). *Waiting for God* (E. Craufurd, Trans.). Harper Perennial Modern Classics.

Winnicott, D. W. (1958). The capacity to be alone. *International Journal of Psychoanalysis*, 39, 416–420.

Winnicott, D. W. (1960). The theory of the parent-infant relationship. *International Journal of Psychoanalysis*, 41, 585–595.

Winnicott, D. W. (1965). *The maturational processes and the facilitating environment: Studies in the theory of emotional development*. Hogarth Press and the Institute of Psycho-Analysis.

Winnicott, D. W. (1967). The place where we live. *International Journal of Psycho-Analysis*, 48, 386–391.

Winnicott, D. W. (1969). The use of an object and relating through identifications. In *Playing and Reality* (pp. 86–94). Routledge.

Winnicott, D. W. (1971). *Playing and reality*. Tavistock Publications.

Winnicott, D. W. (1974). Fear of breakdown. *International Review of Psycho-Analysis*, 1, 103–107.

Winnicott, D. W. (1975). Birth memories, birth trauma, and anxiety. *The International Psycho-Analytical Library*, 100, 174–193. (Original work published 1949).

# Index

Note: Locators in **bold** refer **tables** and locators followed by "n" refer end notes.

For Product Safety Concerns and Information please contact our EU representative GPSR@taylorandfrancis.com
Taylor & Francis Verlag GmbH, Kaufingerstraße 24, 80331 München, Germany

www.ingramcontent.com/pod-product-compliance
Ingram Content Group UK Ltd.
Pitfield, Milton Keynes, MK11 3LW, UK
UKHW022014111026
476504UK00011B/416
* 9 7 8 1 0 4 1 3 4 0 5 0 8 *